LIFE IN THE BALANCE

James C. Hefley

While this book is designed for your personal enjoyment and profit, it is also intended for group study. A Leader's Guide with Victor Multiuse Transparency Masters is available from your local bookstore or from the publisher at $2.50.

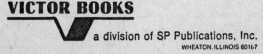

VICTOR BOOKS

a division of SP Publications, Inc.

WHEATON. ILLINOIS 60187

Offices also in Fullerton, California • Whitby, Ontario, Canada • Amersham-on-the-Hill, Bucks, England

Recommended Dewey Decimal Classification: 261:83
  Suggested Subject Headings: CHRISTIAN ETHICS; ETHICS; CONSCIENCE

Library of Congress Catalog Card Number: 79-67854
  ISBN: 0-88207-797-x

VICTOR BOOKS
a division of SP Publications, Inc.
P.O. Box 1825 Wheaton, Illinois 60187

CONTENTS

FOREWORD

Life in the Balance is a forum. As such, it does not make conclusive statements about the issues discussed.

The purpose of this book is to stimulate thought, generate discussion, and motivate you in two ways—to obtain more information about the subjects, and to search out biblical answers which will guide you in making decisions about these life-and-death matters.

The Publisher

INTRODUCTION

The nightmarish future which George Orwell and Aldous Huxley fantasied is closer than we think. No one is laughing now at the idea of babies hatched in state nurseries and electronic behavior modification practiced by a "Ministry of Love" as Orwell suggested in his book *1984*. The *Brave New World* which Huxley imagined in the 25th century is sounding more and more like the late 20th century.

In this "brave new world" there are no absolute norms, no eternal foundations, no spiritual dimensions to human nature. God is only an emanation of physical and chemical processes in man's mind. Man is only the product of evolution, a creature of chance, alone in the universe, who, as psychologist Erich Fromm said, "must become his own source of comfort."

The idea of man becoming a god has not changed. But the content today is different, vastly different, and it will affect all of us, our children, and our children's children.

As Christians, as people who care about God's revelation and man's condition, how will we face the biorevolution?

—Can we ignore it and pull back into our "ghettos" of spiritual fellowship while we await the return of the Lord and the Final Judgment?

—Can we condemn the entire scientific and medical establishment for challenging long-cherished beliefs and tampering with mysteries reserved for God?

—Or will we face the new biotechnical issues squarely? This is the hardest road, but it is the only right alternative. We are citizens of an earthly kingdom too. We should support humanitarian endeavors, while opposing unethical practices and experimentation.

Confronting these issues is the purpose of this book. Six crucial topics are examined, beginning with the startling new variations in human reproduction and concluding with the dilemmas which medical science has placed around dying. Between birth and death, we will consider abortion, genetic engineering, brain research and therapies, and homosexuality.

Two chapters explore each topic. The first is explanatory, the second, interpretative. An exposition of what is happening in the light of science, the Bible, and human needs is presented first. Then a panel of evangelical doctors, scientists, and a few theologians react. They will not always agree, nor will some of their ideas please every reader, but they should be heard respectfully, with further guidance sought through Bible study, prayer, and counsel from other informed Christians.

This book plows new ground for an evangelical Sunday School publisher. Hopefully, it will make us better servants of God in the world in which we live and better witnesses of His awesome sovereignty and matchless love.

I want to express my personal appreciation to the many professional people who so generously shared their experiences and opinions about these sensitive subjects. This book could not have been written without their help.

James C. Hefley

MAJOR CONSULTANTS

Anderson, V. Elving, Ph.D., Professor of Human Genetics at the University of Minnesota and Director of the Dight Institute of Human Genetics.

Buzzard, Lynn R., Executive Director, Christian Legal Society, Oak Park, Illinois.

Esau, Truman, M.D., Psychiatrist and Director of Old Orchard Hospital for the Mentally Ill, Skokie, Illinois.

Grady, John L., M.D., Family Physician, Benton, Tennessee. Formerly Chairman of the Department of Obstetrics and Chief of Staff, Glades General Hospital, Belle Glade, Florida.

Herrmann, Robert L., Ph.D., Professor and Chairman, Department of Biochemistry, Oral Roberts University Schools of Medicine and Dentistry, Tulsa, Oklahoma.

Lester, Lane P., Ph.D., Geneticist, President of Orange Counseling Center, Orlando, Florida; and Southeastern Representative of Institute for Creation Research.

Lindsell, Harold, Ph.D., Theologian; Editor Emeritus of *Christianity Today*.

Mackay, Donald, Ph.D., Brain Physiologist and Professor of Communications at Keel University in England.

Monroe, Thomas C., Jr., M.D., Obstetrician and Gynecologist, East Ridge, Tennessee, and Associate Professor, University of Tennessee Center for Health Sciences and Clinical Education in Chattanooga.

Rawlings, Maurice, M.D., Specialist in Cardiovascular Diseases, Chattanooga, Tennessee, and Associate Professor at the University of Tennessee Center for Health Sciences and Clinical Education in Chattanooga.

Veith, Roger, M.D., Neurosurgeon, Chattanooga, Tennessee.

Weiss, A. Kurt, Ph.D., Professor of Physiology, University of Oklahoma School for Health Sciences, Oklahoma City, Oklahoma.

Wenger, Carl, M.D., General Surgeon, Little Rock, Arkansas, and Associate Professor at the University of Arkansas Medical School.

1

Cloning, Test-Tube Babies and Artificial Insemination

How times have changed! Our grandparents spoke of pregnancy as being "in a family way." Most babies were delivered at home—Jimmy Carter is the first U.S. president to have been born in a hospital. By the time the doctor or granny woman arrived, the other children had been shooed off to stay with relatives. Problems in human reproduction were personal and never discussed in mixed company.

Sex and pregnancy still probably wouldn't match the weather and taxes as general conversation topics. Yet some Christians speak of low sperm counts, blocked fallopian tubes, and breech deliveries with a frankness that would have made an older generation turn crimson.

One of the last medical-sexual taboos to fall is artificial insemination and related practices. Once kept so supersecret that the local obstetrician often didn't know his patient had been inseminated by a fertility specialist, artificial insemination is now being pushed into the open by stories in the public media about more daring means of human conception and development. We're hearing about *test-tube babies* fertilized in the lab and the embryo then implanted in the uterus of the mother; *host mothers* who carry other women's babies to term for a fee (rent-a-womb service); *artificial uterus* where babies may develop in a synthetic environment; and *cloning*—single parent reproduction.

Artificial Insemination

Artificial insemination has been controversial since the first known instance of it, almost 200 years ago. The latest advances and experiments in human biology are even more controversial. Do these "improved" ideas for making babies fall within the divine command to "be fruitful and multiply"? (Gen. 1:28) Are the breathtaking new lab experiments complementary to God's purposes? Could the bioscientists be going beyond what God intended, perhaps be "playing God"? Should Christians be involved? Are there dangers that man could create a race of genetically subhuman creatures? Should there be controls on experiments with human egg cells, sperm, and embryos?

Before attempting to answer these disturbing questions, we will examine the procedures now inciting so much trepidation on one hand and enthusiasm on the other. Artificial insemination (AI) is man's first successful attempt to produce children when the husband cannot fertilize his wife's ovum.

From 10 to 20 thousand AI babies are born in the U.S. each year and many times that number abroad. From one to five hundred thousand AI children are now alive in the U.S. Only a general estimate can be made because of secrecy and minimal record keeping by doctors who strive to protect the privacy of their patients.

Human AI is basically no different from the procedure long used by domestic animal breeders. Live male sperm is inseminated into the female uterus where conception occurs. About half of all U.S. dairy cows are conceived this way. Only the finest purebred bulls are used, with their sperm frozen and banked until ready for shipment to farms. Milk yield of these scientifically bred bovines is a proven 65 percent higher than from cows conceived from uncontrolled breeding. Corresponding upgrading is noted in beef cattle, horses, and other animals.

The first authenticated successful human insemination occurred in

1790 when Dr. John Hunter so enabled the wife of a London linen merchant to have a child. The first American AI children were born in 1866. Today the procedure is routinely done by hundreds of gynecologists and human fertility specialists.

The woman comes to the physician's office at her time of ovulation. He painlessly inserts part of the sperm sampling with a syringe, places a plastic pessary containing the remainder in her vagina, and instructs her to leave it there for six or eight hours. If conception results she begins her regular schedule of visits to her obstetrician. If not, she returns for another attempt. On the average about three inseminations are required for pregnancy.

1. Husband. AIH (artificial insemination husband) accounts for only a small percentage of AI pregnancies. The husband may have fertile sperm; yet for physical or psychological reasons, paralysis for example, he is unable to participate in normal coitus. He might be going off to war, about to have a vasectomy, or soon undergo prostate surgery which could render him sterile. Sperm can be taken by masturbation and inseminated in his wife, or frozen and kept for a later date. Or he may have a low sperm count. In this case the doctor takes several specimens which he concentrates for a successful insemination.

There are no legal questions about AIH. Only Roman Catholics and Orthodox Jews make religious objections to certain types of AIH. For most couples, it is a recommended method of having a child when the standard way is not possible.

2. Donor. AID (artificial insemination donor) is the same, except that a second man provides the sperm. Legal and moral complexities abound. In only 14 states is the husband recognized as the legal father of a child born from insemination of another man's seed. State courts have given contradictory opinions in cases where child custody and/or support is involved. In 1955, the Superior Court of Cook County (Chicago) ruled: "With or without the consent of the husband, 'AID' is contrary to public policy and good morals, and constitutes adultery on the part of the mother. A child so conceived is not born in wedlock and therefore is illegitimate." New York and California courts have said that where the husband gives his consent, the AID child is legitimate. Oklahoma law is considered a model by AID proponents. There a couple requesting AID simply go before a judge and sign consent papers as if they were adopting a child.

Upon learning that they cannot have children, a couple desiring AID may ask their local doctor or pastor for guidance. The counselor will refer them to a specialist who can perform the insemination. Because of feared legal problems and disapproval of the families, many couples visit out-of-town specialists surreptitiously. Then when the wife becomes pregnant, she goes to her own doctor for delivery. Unknowingly, he attests that the husband is the true father. AID practitioners admit that this is often done, but say they must respect the couple's desire for secrecy. Dr. S.J. Behrman of Royal Oak, Michigan, who has inseminated hundreds of women, says, "Laws are desperately needed to get us all—doctor, donor, patient and child—out from under a cloud."

The moral and religious questions are equally formidable.

- Is it right to parent a child whose legitimacy is in question?
- Is it proper to allow a doctor to name the husband as the father, when he is not?
- Will an AID child help or hurt a marriage?
- Is AID another form of adultery?
- Does AID fall within God-ordained procreation in marriage?
- What about the moral responsibilities of the donor and doctor?
- Would a couple be better advised to try to adopt a child?

The first question is not relevant in the 14 states where AID children are legitimate. The last question is not as pertinent as it once was. Abortions and the number of unwed mothers who now decide to keep their children have markedly reduced the chances of adoption. Unless a couple is willing to take an older child, or one that is severely handicapped, an AID baby may be their only hope.

The other questions demand thoughtful consideration. The Bible certainly forbids lying and deception. "Lying lips are an abomination to the Lord. . . . A false witness will not go unpunished" (Prov. 12:22; 19:5). "Do not lie to one another," Paul exhorted Christians, "since you laid aside the old self with its evil practices" (Col. 3:9).

Can a man "father" a child other than biologically? He can certainly be a father to an adopted child. Can he likewise "father" an AID child, when he has freely consented to the insemination and shared the burden and joy of developing life with his spouse? The answer to this question depends on the latitude one gives fatherhood.

The few surveys made of AID marriages indicate that such couples have a much lower divorce rate than the general population. Dr. Sheldon Payne of the Shelton Clinic in Los Angeles has determined that only 10 percent of his patients later divorce, compared to a rate of over 50 percent in the state at large. This low rate is attributed to careful screening of applicants and the maturity of the couples when they come to the clinic.

Does AID constitute adultery? Religious leaders are greatly divided here. Catholic theologians who follow official dogma say Yes. Explains Father Francis L. Filias, S.J., Chairman of the Department of Theology at Loyola University in Chicago: "It (AID) violates the marriage bond in which husband and wife have a right to each other's lifegiving powers." Father Filias believes that a husband "cannot give away his God-given right to his wife's procreative powers."

Conservative and Reformed Jewish rabbis and officials of the Lutheran Church of America and the United Presbyterian Church disagree with the Catholic position. A United Presbyterian committee said: "To discover in artificial insemination by an anonymous donor an act of adultery is certainly to give the word a meaning that it does not have in the New Testament" (Time, June 1, 1962).

Many evangelicals tend to agree. "It depends on the personal preference of the couple," says Dr. Wallace Denton, director of the Marriage Counseling Center at Purdue University and a Southern Baptist lay leader. David Mains, director of the Chapel of the Air radio ministry, does not see this as adultery. "While the husband doesn't directly participate in physical intercourse, neither does the donor. If my wife and I couldn't have children normally, I don't think I would object." "Lustful desire is the essential point of adultery," according to Dr. V. Elving Anderson, geneticist and Baptist General Conference layman. "The Old Testament Levirate marriage law provided in essence for donor insemination when it obligated a near kinsman of a deceased man to father an heir for the widow."

Of procreation in marriage, the psalmist declared, "Behold, children are a gift of the Lord; the fruit of the womb is a reward. Like arrows in the hand of a warrior, so are the children of one's youth. How blessed is the man whose quiver is full of them" (Ps. 127:3-5). Does a child conceived from another man's bequest belong in a husband's "quiver"? The Bible doesn't explicitly answer this, or many other medical-ethical dilemmas which trouble society today.

Doctors identify the typical donor as a medical student or hospital resident who is paid about $30 for his contribution. Genesis 38:9-10, which states that God was displeased when Onan spilled his seed on the ground, is sometimes applied to an AID donor. But the context indicates that God was displeased by Onan's refusal to impregnate his deceased brother's wife and "raise up seed" for him.

While many donors apparently never have second thoughts, Dr. Denton recalls one anxious Jewish student who confided that he had been asked to donate for insemination. " 'I worry,' he told me, 'about meeting children on the street and wondering if one might be mine.' "

Some doctors will not do artificial insemination. While Dr. J.J. Gold of Chicago has helped many wives become pregnant with their husbands' sperm, he declines to do AID because of the many problems involved. However, none of the doctors interviewed for this chapter think that AID is implicitly immoral.

A new cloud over AID doctors concerns insemination of single women. On March 16, 1976, The Chicago Sun-Times reported that a University of Wisconsin survey of 379 physicians administering AID turned up 47 who admitted inseminating single women, some of whom were lesbians. There are no laws to prevent this, but children born could suffer social stigma in future years. Furthermore, it is immoral for a woman to conceive a child outside of sanctioned marriage.

Where married couples are involved, AID doctors select donors to match the husband's physical appearance (hair, skin, eye color, height, build, blood type, etc.). The University of Wisconsin study also showed that some doctors even take medical histories of donor families as a precaution against inherited diseases. Other doctors do not and only 12 percent of the physicians answering the questionnaire said they did chromosome tests on donors to prevent birth of a Down's syndrome (mongoloid) child. Only 30 percent checked for traits that might result in sickle-cell anemia, diabetes, and other defects. Failure of doctors to test donors for genetic diseases borders on irresponsibility, especially when AID is sought because the husband is a carrier of a genetic affliction.

The survey revealed that over two thirds of the AID physicians were failing to keep any files on donors. Some of those who did were using the same donor for a number of pregnancies. One donor for six pregnancies was not unusual and in one instance, a single donor had "fathered" 50 children. This raises the specter of half brothers and sisters unknowingly marrying one another and possibly producing defective offspring.

Doctors with large AID practices tend to keep better records and used sperm banks. Some banks are computerized for quick screening. It is not extraordinary to use one or two-year-old sperm. Other studies have shown that sperm does not lose its potency with limited aging. A University of Arkansas researcher discovered that a group of 3000 children, conceived with thawed donor sperm, suffered only one sixth of the birth defects found in newborns as a whole.

The computerized sperm banks worry Father Filias, the Loyola University theologian quoted earlier. "The sperm bank is the scientist gone mad and the scientist gone mad plays God," he says. "This is an area that God does not intend to be in our power."

Test-Tube Babies

In vitro fertilization (IVF) of an egg outside the mother's body was the next logical step beyond artificial insemination.

IVF experiments date to the 1940s when Dr. John Rock of Harvard, father of the birth control pill, took eggs from female cancer patients, mixed them with sperm in a test tube, and brought them to a three-cell stage. About a decade later, Dr. Landrum Shettles of Columbia University grew fertilized embryos in a lab culture to 16 cells.

In Italy in 1959, Daniele Petrucci announced he had sustained an IVF human embryo for 29 days. He had ended the experiment because the embryo "had become deformed and enlarged, a monstrosity." Dr. Petrucci was accused of murder by some Catholic clergy and pressured by the Vatican to grow no more embryos.

Three years later English scientists removed two fertilized eggs from two English sheep, tucked them in the oviduct of a live rabbit, and shipped the hare to South Africa. There the eggs were removed and implanted in two ewes which gave birth to lambs.

More experiments followed and in 1973 International CryoBiological Services, Inc. of St. Paul, Minnesota reported "bovine ova transfer." Eggs were taken from "high quality cows," fertilized with sperm from superior bulls, and the embryos implanted in "less valuable incubator cows" for development until birth.

In 1971 Dr. Shettles removed an egg from a woman with diseased fallopian tubes, fertilized it with her husband's sperm, and implanted the embryo into the uterus of a second woman. Two days later when the recipient underwent a previously scheduled hysterectomy, the embryo was found to have multiplied into several hundred cells.

In 1974 Douglas Bevis stunned the British Medical Association by claiming the birth of three babies which he had fertilized in the lab and implanted back into their mothers' wombs. Since Bevis refused to identify the participants, doctors doubted his story.

One of the doubters was Dr. Patrick Steptoe who was then working on the process with his partner, Dr. Robert Edwards. In 1978 they presented Baby Louise Brown, "the world's first test-tube baby." The mother had previously been unable to conceive because her fallopian tubes were irreversibly blocked. A second such baby has been born in Scotland. More are on the way, with the scientists reporting a 10 percent success rate of achieving pregnancies. Enterprising businessmen are now capitalizing on the publicity. One advertises "test-tube baby plants" for sale.

Controversy in the U.S. had been building before the Steptoe-Edwards' achievement. Dr. James Watson, the U.S. Nobel Prize biologist, told a congressional subcommittee that a "test-tube" baby would be produced and warned that chaos "will break loose, politically and morally, all over the world." That didn't quite happen. Steptoe and Edwards received worldwide acclaim from their colleagues. For example, the American Fertility Society meeting in San Francisco gave Steptoe an ovation after he presented a lecture on his work.

Fears of where IVF might lead stopped U.S. grants in 1975. After the English triumph, the Ethics Advisory Board of the Department of Health, Education, and Welfare held hearings. Protestant moral theologian Paul Ramsey warned of possible physical and psychological damage to IVF children. Bishop Thomas Kelly, general secretary of the National Conference of Catholic Bishops urged that the ban be continued.

But after several scientists defended IVF, the board recommended that HEW lift the ban with certain qualifications: The public must be told of any evidence that IVF produces a higher number of abnormal fetuses. Embryos can only be formed from sperm and eggs of "lawfully married couples." Experimentation must be done only during the first 14 days after fertilization, the time required for normal implantation of an embryo in the womb.

Artificial Wombs

Scientists are now working on artificial wombs to aid infant "preemies" likely to die from breathing difficulties caused by hyaline membrane disease. Twenty-five thousand preemies die each year in the U.S. from this affliction. Duplicating the amniotic sac and fluid in which a baby develops in a mother's womb is enormously difficult. There are problems with exchanging gases, liquids, solids, and hormones between the fetus and its prenatal environment.

Soviet scientists are way ahead with research on an artificial womb. After the crackdown by the Vatican on his work in Italy, Dr. Petrucci gave his knowledge to the Russians. They reportedly now have about 250 human fetuses growing in artificial wombs at the Institute of Experimental Biology in Moscow. One "human" form is said to have been kept alive for six months, and a rabbit sustained all the way to birth. The Russians have declined to show even pictures of their products. Western scientists suspect gross abnormalities.

Gynecologists expect IVF to be as available in a few years for women who cannot conceive normally as AID is now for those whose husbands cannot impregnant them with potent sperm. There will likely be "host mothers" advertising their wombs for hire in classified ads. Egg banks will develop alongside sperm banks. Futurists predict that a couple or a single woman will be able to go to a "parent store" and select a frozen embryo with the genetic traits desired. Some say there will even be embryo implants in males, with babies delivered by cesarean section.

Artificial wombs will be for those who want a complete laboratory product.

Cloning

The end is not yet in sight. Some think human cloning will be next, the asexual reproduction of genetically identical humans without egg or sperm from the opposite sex. *Cloning*, from a Greek word for "off-shoot" or "twig," has long been a standard practice of horticulturists. The real excitement came in 1961 when Dr. J.B. Gurdon of Oxford University cloned a frog. A Massachusetts scientist, Dr. Audrey Muggleton-Harris now has a U.S. grant to clone a mouse.

To grasp how cloning works, we need to understand first the genetic order in normal bisexual reproduction. The female egg and male sperm each contributes 23 chromosomes to the first cell of new life. The chromosomes are comprised of genes, which are made of chemical DNA (deoxyribonucleic acid), the fundamental component of living tissue and the blueprint of life. The cell with its 46 chromosomes divides and redivides into additional cells, each containing 46 new chromosomes, identical to the first set. The baby thus inherits a mixed genetic ancestry from two parents and their ancestries. This provides for almost limitless genetic variation and makes every person physically unique.

For the frog cloning, Dr. Gurdon removed an unfertilized egg cell from a South African clawed frog and destroyed its nucleus with ultraviolet radiation. He then plucked a body cell, containing a full set of chromosomes, from the intestinal wall of another frog. He removed and transplanted the nucleus of this cell into the egg cell which he put back in the first frog's body. Tricked into thinking it was properly fertilized, the converted egg developed into an identical twin of its single parent, the donor of the nucleus.

Cloning will be much more difficult for humans. For one thing, a human egg cell is much smaller than a frog cell. Even if a body cell nucleus could be transferred to an egg cell, chemical incompatibilities might be too great to overcome or the fusion could produce an indescribably abnormal fetus. Dr. Steptoe and many scientists say human cloning is impossible. Others think differently. Dr. Paul Segal, a microbiologist at the University of California at Berkeley, forecasts the first human clone in 10 to 20 years.

Enthusiasts see cloning as a way to reproduce genius. "We can always use additional Einsteins, Picassos, Beethovens, or Tolstoys," says science writer Isaac Asimov, an atheist. "If such great people have children in the ordinary way, there chromosomes are mixed with those of their mates and the combination may not represent quite the genius of the one parent. If we clone genius, on the other hand, we have new individuals with the precise chromosomes of that genius" (*Family Weekly,* March 4, 1979, pp. 4-5). The damper, Asimov concedes, is that human beings are not the product of chromosomes alone, but also of different eras and environments.

Cloning is further seen as a way to provide models for medical experiments. One proposal is to clone domestic servants. Another is that clones might provide extra organs or limbs when transplants are needed. Presumably, this would solve the rejection problem presently encountered in transplant surgery. Still another idea is that one's brain cells might be frozen at death and preserved until reconstruction becomes possible through cloning. Science writer Robert Wilson did this for his 16-year-old daughter Luna, a murder victim.

Could clones function as ordinary people? They would be the same as identical twins, produced from a single fertilized egg. Even if placed in different environments, they would, as identical twins, have many similarities. For example, identical twins James E. Lewis and James A. Spring of Ohio recently met after being separated for 40 years by adoption. Both had named their dogs "Toy." Both had trained in law enforcement. Both enjoyed similar hobbies: blueprinting, drafting, and carpentry. Both had married first wives named Betty. Both named their first sons James Allan. They were physically alike except for hairstyles. Even their brainwaves and heartbeat patterns were the same. What would it be like for 100 identical children to grow up together in the same community?

Warnings

None of this is purely science fiction. It is being seriously predicted as something that could happen. As expected, warning signals are being raised by theologians as well as scientists.

Dr. Leon Kass of the Kennedy Institute and principal author of a National Academy of Science assessment of biotechnology, warns:

"What is new about embryo transfer is a divorce of the generation of new life from human sexuality and ultimately from the confines of the human body. Sexual intercourse will no longer be needed for generating new life. This novelty leads to two others: There is a new co-progenitor, the embryologist-geneticist-physician; and there is a new home for generation, the laboratory. The mysterious and intimate processes of generation are to be moved from the darkness of the womb to the bright (fluorescent) light of the laboratory" (Richard M. Restak, *Premeditated Man,* The Viking Press, pp. 63-64).

Dr. Kass believes that "One can purchase quality control of the product only by the depersonalization of the process. Is there not wisdom in the mystery of nature that joins the pleasure of sex, the communication of love, and the desire for children in the very activity by which we continue the chain of human existence? Is not human procreation, if properly understood and practiced, itself a humanizing experience?" (*The Chicago Tribune,* July 30, 1972, p. 24)

This National Academy of Sciences scholar is also concerned about human female eggs removed for embryo transfer. He wonders what happens to the eggs not chosen. "Would they ever be used . . . on another woman, for instance, whose eggs turned out to be less than optimum? Or are they discarded? If so, this is a distinctly different situation than prevails in abortion. The embryos discarded here are wanted, at least for a while. They are deliberately created, used for a time, and then deliberately destroyed. I am concerned about the effects and the attitude toward and respect for human life engendered in persons engaged in these practices. . . . Shall we leave it so that discarding laboratory-grown embryos is a matter solely between a doctor and his plumber?" (Restak, *Premeditated Man,* p. 65)

Professor Norman Anderson, a renowned English lawyer-theologian and frequent lecturer to evangelical students, is negative toward all procedures involved in producing children outside of the union of man and wife. "The very idea of the selective breeding of human beings in the manner of race horses or prize cattle seems to me to constitute a fundamental degradation of man made in the image of God. . . . This brings us back to the principle of . . . the 'creation ordinance' of the basic institution of marriage and family relationships; and just as sex, for the

Christian, must (for this reason among others) be confined to marriage, so too, it seems to me, should the conception of a child" *Issues of Life and Death,* InterVarsity Press, pp. 51-52).

When asked, "Does the Scripture shed any light on the subject of artificial insemination?" Billy Graham answered:

"The procreative process was devised by an infinite, wise God, and is treated as most sacred in the Scriptures. . . . The Scriptures mention no other method of reproduction of the human species, and . . . any deviation from the normal method which God ordained has no scriptural basis. Of course, artificial insemination was unknown in the days when the Bible was written, but even so, there is a shadow of doubt present when the Scriptures are silent" (*Billy Graham Answers,* Newspaper Column).

Evangelical theologian Carl Henry sees the issue as symbolic of man's failure in the Garden of Eden. "Adam's eating of the Edenic tree of knowledge without moral sanction and ethical commitment cost him spiritual life. The temptation is now commonplace to devour the fruit of the tree of knowledge in order to become like gods. . . . We are here faced again with the crisis of Eden: We want to touch the tree of knowledge, quite indifferently to God's consent and purpose. . . . It may precipitate the destruction of the very civilization and culture that some spokesmen for science had only a few generations ago hoped to lift to the brink of utopia" (*Journal of the American Scientific Affiliation,* September, 1978, p. 99).

Still there are Christian authorities who have few fears, so long as the experiments are controlled by moral guidelines. They see IVF, like AID, as another means of helping desperate couples have children. Dr. Donald Mackay, the famous English brain physiologist and lecturer to many evangelical faculties, calls IVF "trivial" in respect to morality. The only question, he thinks, is the stewardship of time devoted to producing more children in an already overpopulated world. Nor is he unduly alarmed about cloning. You will see further comments by Dr. Mackay in the following chapter.

Some scientists think too much attention is being given to man's accomplishments in the laboratory. Dr. Lewis Thomas, for example, president and chief executive officer of Memorial Sloan-Kettering Cancer Center in New York, wonders in his book *The Medusa and the Snail* (The Viking Press), why so much fuss was made over the test-tube baby. The true miracle, he declares, has always been the union of egg and sperm and the emergence of a cell that can develop into a human being. "The mere existence of that cell," he says, "should be one of the greatest astonishments of the earth. People ought to be walking around all day . . . calling to each other in endless wonderment, talking of nothing except that cell." Dr. Thomas declares, "No one has the ghost of idea how this works, and nothing else in life can ever be so puzzling" (review in *Time,* May 14, 1979, p. 88).

2

Christian Perspectives on Cloning, Test-Tube Babies, and Artificial Insemination

DR. LANE P. LESTER, HUMAN GENETICIST

Dr. Lester doesn't consider AID immoral. "Adultery is a physical act. AID does introduce a third party into a marriage, but the procedure is reproductive and nonphysical in that there is no union as in intercourse.

"All of God's commandments for man make good sense. The prohibition against adultery makes psychological sense. The command against incest makes good sense for biological reasons. Artificial insemination is, of course, not mentioned in the Bible, but when a third party is involved, I can see that for psychological reasons it could cause real problems.

"Host mothers," he says, "will probably multiply given society's trend away from any kind of real spiritual morality, and toward humanistic philosophy.

"While cloning of humans makes good science fiction at this time, I don't think it's been done. It may be technically possible, but I believe the pressures of society will prevent it.

"If something can be done, there is some scientist who would like to do it. There is quick fame for doing something outstanding. With rapid transmission of information through the media, a person can get a worldwide reputation overnight if he does something startling. That wasn't possible years ago.

"I don't pretend to be an expert in cloning. It's been done with frogs and I expect it can be done with mice. Laboratory mice, you might say, are genetically pure. The harmful mutations have been substantially bred out. But the human is full of harmful mutations, genetic mistakes that happened over the history of the human species. If you began doubling that in cloning, all of a sudden millions of mutant genes would be present in two doses. That's all it takes to cause disease from many of these genetic mutations. It would almost certainly be lethal. But I wouldn't be at all surprised if someone has tried it. It's just another way man thinks he can improve the species.

"As Christians we need to become better informed and test these ideas and proposed techniques against Christian understanding of the Scriptures to see if they violate God's principles. Although I'm pessimistic as to how much good Christians can accomplish, I know we can do something. That was proven recently in Florida when Christians banded together and helped defeat casino gambling."

DR. ELVING ANDERSON, HUMAN GENETICIST

"The so-called test-tube baby," Dr. Anderson says, "was not unexpected. There were certain technical problems, but they were not all that tremendous."

He suspects, however, that few of the women who will want to conceive babies by the Steptoe-Edwards' procedure will be able to. This is not just because of the difficulty in finding a doctor who can do the job, but due to mishaps which occur in ordinary conceptions and early prenatal development.

"In apparently normal conceptions," he says, "about half do not succeed. Two of six will terminate before the mother knows anything about it. In known pregnancies, one of six will terminate in a natural miscarriage.

"There are some random elements that occur in the process of forming the zygote (the initial cell of new life). Changes in chromosomes can be attributed to this. About one of three natural or spontaneous abortions involve serious chromosomal changes or errors. Most of these are lethal to the fetus and cause the miscarriage. The process of conception and prenatal development is very complex and things can go wrong. Natural abortions are, in a sense, a way of adjusting to that reality.

"Given these facts and the experimental status of the Steptoe-Edwards' procedure, I expect that the failure rate will continue to be high.

"Ovum transplant to a host, another woman, is not much more difficult than the test tube. This, like artificial insemination by donor, involves a third party, but it isn't quite the same. The woman involved in carrying the child has a much greater investment emotionally than an AID donor who has no emotional or physical attachment.

"I have said that I don't believe AID constitutes adultery. Ovum transplant to a host mother could be adultery only in a very special sense. It carries none of the social, psychological, or emotional components of adultery."

Regarding cloning, Dr. Anderson believes that David M. Rorvik's book on the reality of cloning is a hoax. (*In His Image: The Cloning of a Man,* Lippincott.) "I know of no one in the scientific world who takes it seriously. The book follows all of the author's pet themes in science writing. For example, he had earlier written about decompression as it was used by a doctor in South Africa. During pregnancy the woman would wear an attachment something like an iron lung around her abdominal region for several hours. It was supposed to apply negative pressure. Rorvik includes this as one feature of the birth of the cloned child. But that technique is essentially unused in this country. There are many other features of the book which suggest that it is fiction.

"Cloning," Dr. Anderson emphasizes, "has not been done in mammals yet. So far the problem has been that for mammals, the nucleus of the adult cell is too specialized to be reprogrammed to start the development of an embryo.

"There's nothing wrong with cloning research on experimental animals. I just can't see any reason to do it on humans. Cloning doesn't solve any problem that couldn't be solved in some other way. It doesn't provide any answers to human concerns, misery, pain. In my view, it's of no value.''

DR. THOMAS C. MONROE, OBSTETRICIAN AND GYNECOLOGIST

"We do artificial insemination from husbands and donors right here in our office,'' Dr. Monroe says. ''If the husband wants to inject the donor's sperm, we let him. But we never mix husband and donor sperm. That's foolishness, especially if the husband's sperm is known to be bad. You can't mix good sperm with bad sperm and come out with good sperm.

"As I see it there's no way that AID is adultery. The sperm is obtained by masturbation, for a purpose which is good. I think a Christian could be a donor. Certainly.

"Test-tube baby? It's not test tube at all, it's a nontubal baby. It wasn't conceived in the fallopian tube. It is implanted at the blastocyst stage. To my way of thinking, then it becomes alive.

"I'm all for the nontubal process. A lot of couples will be able to have children who wouldn't otherwise. I think it will be done here in this country with extreme regularity within the next two to five years. If you can produce a baby for parents to raise, to me that is good.

"Cloning humans is ridiculous. There's no way that will ever be. Impossible. Fiction stuff.''

DR. HAROLD LINDSELL, THEOLOGIAN

Dr. Lindsell thinks that the questions being raised now in human biology are ''very difficult, but that this shouldn't keep us from wrestling with them. One needs to ask first, 'What is your source for your ethical and moral principles? Do you have any such principles?'

"Since Scripture teaches that God is the Maker and we know the means by which He has created, I think we should be very careful that we don't try to trespass beyond man's boundaries.

"Some of these recent developments present no problem at all. The Steptoe-Edwards baby is a good example. Here you have a woman who cannot conceive. Her husband's sperm and her egg are brought together outside of the uterus to get a union. The embryo is implanted back in the woman's womb so she can bear life. I see nothing wrong with that. However, I do see a problem if a third party is involved.

"Since I believe that life begins at conception, it does trouble me that some of the implanted embryos have died. Are they true human life? Where do they go? That's like asking where do embryos and fetuses go when they are aborted spontaneously or deliberately. Will they grow and develop as persons in the afterlife? The Bible doesn't specifically answer, but I think they are redeemed by Christ.

"I have no objection whatsoever to cloning of animals. But cloning human beings—well, I have serious reservations.

"It hasn't been done in human beings, and likely never will be. There is the question of whether the soul of man is transmitted through the sexual union of male and female, or whether it is a special, immediate creation. I don't know the answer, but it would have to be considered if human cloning became a reality.

"Somewhere there must be a point of limitation. I wonder if man is not going beyond the boundaries."

DR. DONALD MACKAY, SPECIALIST IN BRAIN PHYSIOLOGY

Dr. MacKay believes science and Christianity need not conflict. "The key to the whole problem of the relation of science to the Christian faith is that God, and God's activity come in not only as extras here and there, but are everywhere. If God is active in any part of the physical world, He is in all. If the divine activity means anything, then *all* the events of what we call the physical world are dependent on that activity" (*The Clockwork Image,* InterVarsity Christian Press, p. 57). In this context, he made the following comments:

"When you ask the question: 'Is there anything off limits for man?' any answer is liable to be misunderstood. I would say that all of us in science function essentially as mapmakers in God's world. In principle, then, it is not just that we have permission, but that we have some *obligation* to get out there and map it so that the people who come after us can use the map.

"Now mapmaking is wrong when it infringes on the moral law. Suppose someone said, 'I'm a psychologist and I would like to study the psychology of adultery. Therefore I have to become an adulterer for the sake of my chosen profession.' That would be nonsense from the biblical point of view. Nobody can pretend that part of our stewardship in God's world requires mapmaking at such a cost.

"Apart from moral considerations, I know of no biblical guidance that prohibits any particular area of research. For example, there are people who say we should never have investigated nuclear energy. That objection is not biblically valid, although it might well be that we should impose more precautions. Nuclear science is simply mapping one more part of God's world—and we may yet have reason to give thanks for the map.

"The test-tube baby is a different matter, because it concerns a particular *application* of knowledge. Although I see nothing immoral about it from the biblical point of view, so long as only married couples are involved, expending resources in this way may not be good stewardship when the world is already bursting with too many people. But perhaps this argument is not compassionate enough for the woman who cannot conceive otherwise.

"Even cloning, as such, does not seem to me to transgress any biblical injunction. I know it's said that cloning would destroy human dignity, but I think this fastens on the wrong target. We all know that it doesn't destroy human dignity for someone to have an identical twin, provided that we use some simple devices, like giving them different names, to let them function as individuals. Logically, I can't see any reason why having 100 'identical twins' would reduce the dignity of any one of them, as long as commonsense precautions prevail.

"But having said this, the objection that I see to cloning is again on grounds of stewardship. Who told us that it would be good long-term stewardship to replenish the earth by reducing the variety of genetic types? Maybe our human gene pool is as good as it is only because of the variety of individuals who contribute to it. To mess with such a delicately balanced system could be disastrously irresponsible. It would also be very difficult to ensure proper psychological development in cloned children deprived of a normal family background.

"What I am saying in general terms is this: Scientific knowledge as such is from God, and is neutral. The proper use of scientific knowledge is our duty to God. But we must look to Him for the wisdom to use it rightly.''

3

Abortion: The Blight of America

Get ready for a global shock! Over 40 million babies were deliberately aborted in 1978, one in every four pregnancies. In the United States alone, a million were put to death, most of them for the convenience of the mother. This brings to six million the number of fetuses deliberately aborted in the U.S. since the Supreme Court struck down restrictive state laws on abortion in 1973. Harold O.J. Brown, chairman of the Christian Action Council, ominously comments: "America has now destroyed more innocent lives through abortion than Hitler did in his extermination chambers" (Open letter, February 20, 1979).

Free abortions, those paid for by taxpayer funds, are available in many states. The University of California at Berkeley provides free abortion counseling and services for about 250 women students every year. Other state universities are expected to follow suit.

Commercial abortion mills advertising pregnancy testing and "counseling" thrive in cities with populations over 100,000. Scores of self-advertised clinics and counseling centers operate in large metropolises such as New York City, where abortions outnumbered births in 1975. Although some people believe these clinics are supposed to be strictly regulated, in actual fact, many are little better than the back-alley butchers who operated before abortion became legal.

In Chicago, a 1979 investigation by two *Sun-Times* reporters uncovered horrendous practices. Counselors were applying high pressure salesmanship. Pregnancy tests were falsified, with doctors performing abortions on nonpregnant women; records of patients' vital signs were altered; and critical lab tests were lost. Many operations were performed by unqualified persons and some patients had to have hysterectomies afterward. But the revenue was good: Doctors performing an abortion every three minutes earned $2,000 an hour. One physician made a pencil mark on the leg of his scrub suit for each abortion, tallying up at the end of the day.

Live Fetuses

Some fetuses are actually aborted alive and sent to a hospital nursery. Other live babies are killed. In a celebrated case, Boston physician Kenneth Edelin was acquitted in a 1977 appeal of charges that he killed a live baby which he aborted by hysterotomy. In 1973, Edelin had been convicted by a lower court on the same charge. The decision of the higher court served notice that doctors need not fear malpractice or criminal prosecution in similar situations.

Shortly after Edelin's acquittal, Dr. William Waddill of Santa Ana, California was asked to abort the 20-week-old fetus of the unwed 18-year-old daughter of a local principal.

The attempted abortion failed and the baby, born alive with apparent brain damage, died shortly thereafter. Dr. Waddill was charged with "wrongful death" of the baby because he did not undertake heroic efforts to save it. And the girl who wanted the abortion is suing the doctor for 17 million dollars for not saving the baby's life! The legal proceedings are still under way.

What if a doctor thinks a fetus can survive and fails to administer life support? Until recently he would have been in trouble. The Supreme Court has ruled that he cannot be prosecuted.

The Stanford University Law Review reports laboratory experiments on aborted live fetuses. Similar stories keep cropping up, but proof is hard to come by. But one grisly practice has stopped. A large New York firm no longer offers in its educational catalog human embryos embedded in plastic.

Infanticide and Euthanasia

Abortion has become one of the most serious problems of our society. No longer is it seen as a last-resort operation, performed to save the life of the mother or to remove a grossly deformed fetus. In our permissive sex-saturated culture, abortion has become a widely accepted form of pregnancy termination at the desire of the mother, who is often urged on by husband, lover, or family. The fetus is seen as less than human, and of little value.

One of the most concerned evangelical physicians is Dr. C. Everett Koop, chief of pediatric surgery at Children's Hospital in Philadelphia. Before the Supreme Court decision in 1973, Dr. Koop predicted that when the U.S. reached a million abortions a year, we would soon also have infanticide, or killing of live children. He now claims that infanticide is "being practiced widely in this country today, that is, the deliberate killing by active or passive means of a child who has been born" (*His,* February, 1979, p. 18).

An article in the *New England Journal of Medicine* substantiated that physicians at the Yale-New Haven Hospital withheld treatment from babies born with physical defects. The deaths of 14 percent of these babies, were "associated with the discontinuance or withdrawal of treatment" (Raymond Duff, October 25, 1973).

There are also fears that abortion on demand will lead to euthanasia for unwanted old people. Theologian Carl Henry asked the Christian Medical Society: "Is the life of a helpless fetus forfeitable simply because the mother wills its death and the parents sense no Good Samaritan obligation to spare it? If so, do the mother and father in principle forfeit any rights of their own when they become senile and their children are disposed to put them out of the way? . . . If we are free to destroy human life and to deny its dignity at one stage, why not at another?"

When Does Life Begin?

The arguments about abortion have always centered around a definition of life at its various stages. Biologically, new life is launched at conception, when the male sperm fertilizes the egg. At this point of creation, the new cell contains a complete genetic blueprint for the growth and development of a new person. Is this embryo sacred and untouchable by human intervention? Or is it merely life in the making, with value lying only in its potential?

The fertilized egg (zygote) divides and multiplies into a cluster of cells. This cluster (blastocyst) moves through the mother's fallopian tubes to become attached to the uterine wall. But about 25 to 38 percent of all blastocysts are spontaneously expelled before this implantation (nidation) occurs. IUD loops and morning-after pills will also prevent implantation. Many doctors believe that these are not contraception, but rather a form of abortion.

The new cells are now specializing, forming the brain, lungs, heart, and other organs. The connection with the uterus becomes the placenta, an organ of blood vessels. A tiny tube, the umbilical cord carries nourishment and oxygen from the mother's blood through the placenta to the embryo and transports waste products back to be disposed of by the mother's body. Because the embryo is wholly dependent on the mother, proponents of elective abortion say the mother has the right to choose whether to continue the pregnancy or have it terminated by abortion. But the new life, as any obstetrician will tell you, is uniquely different from any appendage in the mother's body.

At eight weeks the embryo is classified as a fetus. It is only about an inch long and weighs around 1/28 of an ounce. Yet brain waves show up on an EEG machine and it has all the basic organs and features of a full human being. It floats in a fluid-filled amniotic sac at the end of the umbilical cord. It can twist and turn, even do somersaults. Is it more of a person now than at one day or one week?

By the 28th week, the fetus can probably survive premature birth. Is it now a person? A Miami judge, Dominic Koo, said so in 1978, in finding an alleged traffic violator innocent. The woman defendant had been ticketed for driving by herself in a traffic lane reserved for car pools. She brought a newborn infant to court, telling the judge she was pregnant when cited. Judge Koo found her innocent on grounds a fetus is considered a person. "There were two people in the car," he said.

By the 38th week, give or take a few days, chemicals in the brain of the unborn baby trigger a secretion that stimulates the mother's uterus to contract. The birth canal enlarges and in normal birth the mother's contractions force the new one into the world. A new life is born, no longer absolutely dependent on the mother, but still unable to survive without human nourishment and care. Someone who deliberately kills it will be charged with murder. Would the mother and an abortionist have been equally guilty before God for destroying it before birth?

Right to Kill?

Abortionists assure pregnant women that their rights take precedence over an unborn dependent, and there is no need to suffer from guilt. Ministers and other counselors say it often doesn't work out this way. Dr. E.J. Daniels, a Southern Baptist evangelist, recalls grandmothers coming to him "with haunting memories of abortions." A mother lamented on Mother's Day, "It's hard for me to accept the praise of the children I have when I think of two I decided not to have."

What of the doctor? Traditionally, physicians have taken medicine's ancient Hippocratic Oath, pledging "to preserve life from its conception" and to "give no drug, perform no operation, for a criminal purpose." Some medical schools now delete the oath from graduation ceremonies.

Doctors in private practice, who have convictions against abortions, refuse to perform them. Hospital nurses and doctors in public and private commercial hospitals have less choice, if any. By the time an OB/GYN physician has completed internship and residency at one of these hospitals, he will have assisted in or performed hundreds of abortions. Does this help explain why older doctors tend to be more conservative on abortion than younger physicians who trained after the Supreme Court ruling?

A poll of 2,500 Christian doctors taken in 1974 by the magazine *Christianity Applied* (November, 1974, pp. 33–34) showed that only 40 percent had ever recommended an abortion. However, 80 percent of the

OB/GYN specialists in the poll said they had performed an abortion. Of the 20 percent who had not, almost four of ten had recommended abortions. Only one OB/GYN doctor said he would not counsel an abortion for any reason.

When the OB/GYN physicians were asked on what grounds they could favor abortion, 88 percent cited physical danger to the mother; 69.1 percent, rape; 57.7 percent, incest; 42.4 percent, potential physical or mental abnormality in the child; 37.7 percent, deep emotional trauma; 13.9 percent, demand of the mother; 13 percent, demand of parents if child is a minor. While evangelical physicians are more conservative than doctors with little or no religious commitment, they are more liberal than Catholic doctors who are generally committed to dogma that forbids abortion for any reason.

Means of Abortion

Abortion is no new practice. Archeologists have evidence that mercury was used as an abortifacient as early as 3,000 B.C. An Assyrian manuscript from 1,500 B.C. recommended insertion of acacia tips which form lactic acid when dissolved in water. Some modern contraceptive jellies contain lactic acid.

Modern methods are far more successful and much safer for the pregnant woman. The intrauterine (IUD) loops and "morning after" pills expel the conceptus before it can become attached to the uterine wall. The IUD is more widely used abroad and is prescribed by many missionary doctors. The "morning after" prostagladins are becoming increasingly available in western countries.

Before 12 weeks the embryo or small fetus can usually be suctioned out into a bottle or pulled out by a curette, a sharp, loop-shaped instrument. A fetus over 12 weeks must often be cut, or crushed by forceps, before being removed.

After 14 weeks the abortionist may stimulate labor by inserting a long needle through the uterine wall to withdraw the amniotic fluid, and then replacing it with a saline solution or another chemical. This "salting out" procedure peels away the skin and usually kills the fetus; but occasionally, one is expelled alive.

A cesarean section operation is usually necessary during advanced pregnancy. Many babies can survive this procedure. Most are deliberately killed in the uterus. Those who should come out alive are suffocated in a plastic bag or drowned in a container of formaldehyde. They are then burned or disposed of in the garbage. Human fetuses have been recovered from dumps in some cities. In Los Angeles the Catholic bishop created a furor by displaying several tiny bodies in a church.

Attitudes Toward Abortion in History

Attitudes toward abortion varied greatly in ancient societies. Assyrian law required death by impalement for a woman who aborted herself.

Abortions in the Roman Empire at the time of Jesus were performed routinely, even encouraged. The Greek philosopher Plato thought abortion useful in the ideal state. Aristotle approved it as a method of population control—a reason also given today.

Infanticide of unwanted babies was also sanctioned in ancient Rome and Greece. The early Christians, who saw both abortion and infanticide as murder, rescued abandoned babies from garbage heaps and gave them tender, loving care. The first orphan homes were probably established to care for such infants.

As the church institutionalized, theologians began retreating as they tried to determine when the soul was infused into the fetus, making it an animate human being. Augustine specified 40 days for a male, 80 days for a female. Thomas Aquinas, the most influential Catholic theologian of the Middle Ages, defined the critical moment as "quickening," when the woman felt the fetal movements. After this time abortion was murder.

Not until 1869 did a Catholic pope declare abortion, at any time after conception, to be a grave sin.

Aquinas' doctrine of quickening was incorporated into English common law. This was carried over into colonial America.

There was no legislation on abortion during the first 75 years of independent America. Christian belief in the sacredness of life kept the abortion incidence down until about 1870. Then in the confusion and decadence that followed the Civil War, abortions increased alarmingly. States began enacting laws, prohibiting abortion except when the pregnancy endangered the mother's life.

Modern Attitudes

The influence of biblical Christianity on American life deteriorated further in the 20th century. Secular humanism gained sway in universities. Man was seen as the product of evolution, separated from animals only by his superior intelligence. The sacred aura around fetal life faded as the philosophy that cultural mores and laws must change with society became a guide for many professionals.

After World War II, secularism accelerated in public life while conservative Christianity rebounded. Christian missions, schools, and other evangelical enterprises prospered. A misunderstanding of the biblical doctrine of separation from the world kept effective numbers of evangelicals out of secular professions and government.

Because stringent state laws against abortion were still on the books, proabortionists claimed that thousands of women, desperate for abortions, were being mutilated or killed by back-alley butchers. Newspapers and magazines ground out sad stories of female victims, with statistics that were often grossly exaggerated. Dr. Denis Cavanagh, professor and chairman of the Department of Gynecology and Obstetrics at St. Louis School of Medicine, says there were no more than 240 such deaths per year before 1973.

The first big break for the abortionists came in 1961 when the American Law Institute (ALI) recommended that abortions be permitted where a licensed physician believed there was "substantial risk" that continuance of pregnancy would "impair the physical or mental health of the mother, or that the child would be born with grave physical or mental defects, or that the pregnancy resulted from rape, incest, or other felonious intercourse." Planned Parenthood and the American Civil Liberties Union pushed the ALI proposal. Within a decade 16 states had liberalized their abortion laws.

New York practically allowed abortion on demand. The New York Abortion Counseling Information and Referral Services distributed a million copies of a propaganda booklet on how to have an abortion. Thousands of women from strict states bought package deals (air fare, taxi, and the doctor's fee) for the "New York run." The national media and liberal politicians applauded the eastern haven of refuge for tortured women who were persecuted by barbaric laws in their own states.

New York went from 1,865 to 200,000 legal abortions in one year. The abortion industry became so large and scandalous that the state legislature repealed the new law, offering legislation permitting abortion only to save the life of the mother. However, Governor Nelson Rockefeller vetoed this bill, and the killing continued on an increasing scale.

The dam kept opening as abortionists pushed court suits across the country. It was inevitable that the Supreme Court would rule, and when it did, the verdict was a victory for abortionists. On January 22, 1973 the Court, by a vote of seven-to-two, virtually demolished all restrictive state laws. A state could not prohibit an abortion until a fetus was "viable" or "capable of meaningful life." This was interpreted to mean abortion on demand through the first six months of pregnancy. After that, an abortion was legal if the mother's physical, emotional, or psychological health was at risk. The language was so broad as to permit, in most cases, an abortion up to the time of expected birth.

In a later decision the Court modified the ruling slightly: A state could not be forced to provide abortions from public funds for poor women. Few states have since exercised this option. Most U.S. citizens must pay taxes to finance what some believe to be murder.

Twenty-three evangelically oriented Christian denominations oppose easy abortion. Mainline denominations holding membership in the National Council of Churches have adopted permissive statements. However, Right-to-Life groups inside these denominations are working for change.

As people of the Book, evangelicals seek biblical backing in opposing easy abortion or opposing it totally. Only one Bible passage, Exodus 21:22-24, touches on the loss of fetal life. If a man should "strike a woman with child so that she has a miscarriage, yet there is no further injury, he shall surely be fined as the woman's husband may demand of him; and he shall pay as the judges decide. But if there is any further injury, then you shall appoint as a penalty life for life, eye for eye, tooth for tooth, hand for hand, foot for foot."

The Hebrew text is difficult, leaving room for two possible interpretations. One view makes a distinction between the penalty required for injury to the woman and fetus. Injury to the fetus is punishable only by fine, while injury to the woman calls for "life for life, eye for eye . . ." The second interpretation applies the law of "life for life, eye for eye . . ." to both mother and premature baby. The first would make the fetus of less value than the mother. The second would hold them of equal value.

Antiabortionists believe that stronger evidence can be drawn from Old Testament passages that God is in every phase of fetal development. A favorite is Psalm 139:13-16: "Thou didst form my inward parts; Thou didst weave me in my mother's womb. I will give thanks to Thee, for I am fearfully and wonderfully made. . . . My frame was not hidden from Thee, when I was made in secret, and skillfully wrought. . . . Thine eyes have seen my unformed substance; And in Thy book they were all written, the days that were ordained for me." Three other Old Testament texts frequently cited are Job 31:15; Isaiah 44:24; and Jeremiah 1:5.

In the New Testament only Luke 1:26-56 speaks directly to this theme. When Mary told her cousin Elizabeth that she was pregnant with the Christ Child by the Holy Spirit, Elizabeth felt her baby (John the Baptist) leap in her womb.

Evangelicals who believe that abortion is sometimes permissible note that the Old Testament presents four justifications for taking human life: capital punishment; manslaughter, when a man kills another "unawares"; just wars; and self-defense. They also point to Romans 13:1-7 and 1 Peter 2:13-15 as commanding Christians to obey the laws of government. These seem to be weak arguments for abortion. If abortion is murder, and a violation of the sixth Commandment, then the Christian must disobey man's law to obey God.

Exceptions

The exceptions which many evangelicals allow for abortion divide into two categories, those affecting the mother and her family, and those affecting the future of the child. Where a choice must be made between the life of mother and child, most will say the mother's right to live must come first. Because of advances in medicine and contraceptives, this choice is rarely necessary today.

- Is abortion justified to relieve the emotional trauma of a woman pregnant from rape?
- What if the woman has strong feelings against abortion?
- Will she suffer guilt later?
- And what of society's need for adoptive children? The supply of adoptive babies has dwindled since 1973.

Incest presents both emotional trauma for the woman and the possibility of a child born in poor genetic health. No mother of sound mentality will probably wish to raise a child fathered by its grandfather. But if she can persevere to delivery, again there is the possibility for adoption.

Exceptions relating to the future of the child are often more difficult to decide. One in a hundred newborns will have a genetic disorder. Doctors can usually identify such a disorder in a fetus. They can also tell if the child will be a carrier of genetic disease. The question becomes: Which genetic disabilities call for an abortion, and which do not? There is, for example, a vast difference between Down's syndrome (mongolism) and spinal bifida where the baby is born with an open spine.

Dr. Koop, who has spent his life correcting birth defects, has often publicly stated that under no circumstances should the so-called defective children be aborted. He cites what God told Moses at the burning bush: "Who has made man's mouth? Or who makes the dumb, or deaf, or the seeing, or the blind? Have not I the Lord?" (Ex. 4:11) Says the Philadelphia surgeon: "Whether you or I like it or not, God makes the perfect and also what we would call the imperfect. This is in His sovereign plan. I don't think I should say that God made a mistake and therefore I am going to get rid of this child" (*His*, February 1979, p. 18).

Physicians with convictions like Dr. Koop's note that some of the world's great geniuses were defective at birth or from diseased families. In one family the mother was tubercular, the father syphilitic, one sibling was born blind, another died at birth, another was deaf and dumb, and another also tubercular. The fifth child, who would have been a prime candidate for abortion today, was Ludwig van Beethoven.

Dr. Koop and other skillful pediatric surgeons have proven that severely deformed children can be helped, children who would certainly have died soon after birth had they been born a few years ago. Debbie Fox, for example, was born with 59 physical abnormalities and without a face. She has undergone 57 separate surgical operations. Today she drives a car, plays the harp, and is a source of inspiration for the many disfigured children whom she visits in hospitals. Unfortunately, few families have access to doctors with the skills to help severely defective children.

Legal Alternatives?

The abortion of babies conceived in rape or incest, and of fetuses known to be severely deformed and/or retarded, is not the major problem. It is the flood of abortions for convenience that causes many horrified evangelicals to join with devout Roman Catholics and others in seeking ways to stop this slaughter.

There appear to be only two legal recourses, both of which present worrisome ramifications. A law might be passed by Congress, outlawing abortion with only a few stringent exceptions. A slightly different law might give control of abortion to states. Either way could bring the legislative branch into conflict with the judicial branch and create a grave governmental crisis.

Liberal members of Congress have already felt the heat. Senator Birch Bayh hurt his chance for the Democratic presidential nomination in 1976 when he took a liberal abortion stand. Several senators, known to be liberal on abortion, are targeted for defeat by Right-to-Life anti-abortionists in the 1980 election.

The second legal possibility is an amendment to the Constitution. The amendment would call for a return to pre-1973 policy, prohibiting abortion on demand. Several state legislatures have already passed resolutions asking that Congress present such an amendment to the states for ratification. Many evangelicals, including President Jimmy Carter, oppose this on grounds that the new law would ride roughshod over the rights of unbelievers and also violate separation of church and state as provided in the First Amendment to the Constitution. Proponents for an antiabortion amendment respond that laws against murder have a religious basis in supporting the sacredness of life.

Right-to-Life groups and the distinctly evangelical Christian Action

Council are lobbying hard for some legal alternative. The CAC is specifically "committed to standing for God's righteousness in calling our nation to bring our human laws into harmony with His Divine Law, and to exhibiting His compassion by engendering the human context to support and sustain those who want to obey God and to protect all life." CAC sponsors include theologian Harold O. J. Brown, the chairman, such other evangelical notables as Stuart Briscoe, Harold Lindsell, Ruth Graham, Elisabeth Elliot, Dr. C. Everett Koop, and Edith Schaeffer.

Christian Responses

Beyond efforts to change the law which virtually allows abortion on demand, evangelical leaders say there are other responses which Christians can make:

- Write letters to newspapers protesting abortion.
- Present the biblical case against abortion in Sunday School, preaching, and on Christian broadcasts and telecasts. Expect, however, that the latter may produce opposition from powerful proabortionists. In 1978 the National Broadcasting Company banned a radio sermon by Dr. Oswald Hoffman on "The Lutheran Hour" which upheld the sanctity of human life. The network claimed it presented only one side. A few weeks later, NBC presented a TV news documentary on abortion which right-to-lifers felt was slanted for the other side.
- Provide Christian sex education in the home and church.
- Initiate crisis ministries to pregnant women through local churches and Christian service organizations. Families in the Peninsula Bible Church in Palo Alto, California open their homes to pregnant young women referred by pastors in other communities.
- Oppose sexual permissiveness on television and in other media by writing letters to media owners and advertisers.
- Work for stronger laws against pornography which strikes at all decency and reverence for life.

Dr. Harold O.J. Brown warns that continuance of permissive, widespread abortion in America may call forth God's judgment on our nation.

4

Christian Perspectives on Abortion: The Blight of America

DR. JOHN L. GRADY,
FAMILY PHYSICIAN AND OBSTETRICIAN

Dr. Grady takes a strong, hard line against abortion. He thinks that the reasons for abortion of babies have been greatly overplayed.

"In more than 13 years of obstetrical practice I never lost a mother from any cause. Moreover, during that time at the public hospital where I was a staff member, thousands of babies were delivered and to my knowledge, not a single one was aborted to save a mother's life. Many qualified obstetricians and gynecologists will testify that there are very few instances where the baby actually threatens the life of the mother. With today's advanced medical knowledge, competent physicians, using the latest medical and surgical techniques, can preserve the lives of both mother and baby."

According to Dr. Grady, most abortions are done with regard to the mother's mental health—as high as 97 percent in some states.

"But no one has ever established a cause-and-effect relationship between pregnancy and mental illness. Women who are emotionally unstable get pregnant, but pregnancy is not the cause of their illness. Statistically, there is no increase in mental illness, suicide, or emotional instability among pregnant women. In fact, there is a decrease!

"Dr. John Phelan, instructor in psychiatry, University of Miami School of Medicine, says, 'We hear that abortion is necessary to protect the mental health of the mother, or that unless an abortion is performed a patient will commit suicide. This approach is fallacious and does not stand up under statistical and clinical scrutiny.'

"Dr. Milton Halpern, chief medical examiner of New York City, states that he can, '. . . hardly recall an autopsy on a death by suicide during the last 25 years which revealed pregnancy.'

"The coroner for the city of Birmingham, N.Y. has 'no record of any woman known to be pregnant having committed suicide.'

"There are many cases," Dr. Grady points out, "where the mother has spoken of abortion early in pregnancy and later on has confessed her gratitude to the physician for not having performed the abortion. It is a fact that most women who have been unhappy to find they were pregnant have been most happy with the baby that resulted from that pregnancy. On the other hand, I have studied case histories of married women who have become troubled, consumed with guilt, and developed significant psychiatric problems following, and because of, abortion. I believe it can be stated with certainty that abortion causes more deep-seated guilt, depression, and mental illness than it ever cures."

What of rape, incest, illegitimacy? Dr. Grady believes, "The baby's right to live outweighs the license of a parent, doctor, or any other individual to exterminate it. Even when there is a social crime perpetrated upon the girl, as in the case of rape, the unborn child is an innocent human being, and in no way responsible for the offense, and should not be punished for the crime or misjudgment of either parent. Throughout history pregnant women, who for one crime or another were sentenced to die, were given a stay of execution until after the delivery of the child. It was the contention of the courts that one could not punish the innocent child for the crime of the mother.

"Pregnancy from rape is very uncommon. Pregnancy occurs on the average of once in every 250-350 acts of intercourse. In rape, pregnancy occurs even less often due to the stress factor. Thus, a highly emotional issue has been made of a statistically rare problem.

"No one denies that it is unfortunate when pregnancy occurs in the single girl, the young, the mentally retarded, and those cases where a baby is simply not wanted, such as the poor with large families or in areas of alleged population explosion. But can a woman eradicate the fetus for her personal convenience because a pregnancy is not wanted? Many of our greatest individuals resulted from unexpected or unwanted pregnancies. Indeed the majority of us living today were not planned or eagerly anticipated.

"What of the rights of the unborn? Will we now reverse the precedents in our law which have held that an infant in the uterus is a person under the law, and does have rights—property rights, recourse for damages, and basic inherent constitutional rights? The Declaration of Independence and the Constitution in the 14th Amendment clearly state that 'All men are endowed by their Creator with certain inalienable rights . . . life, liberty and the pursuit of happiness,' and that 'No state shall make or enforce any law which shall . . . deprive any person of life, liberty, or property without due process of law.' In abortion, who represents the unborn child? Where is his defense attorney? Where is his due process of law, including the right to appeal his sentence of extermination?

"We hear much for the mother's right. Some contend that the mother alone should have the right to determine how many babies she will have. This argument is erroneous because it completely excludes the husband from having any interest or privilege in establishing the family size. And the argument is irrelevant because it substitutes birth control for abortion, and confuses the issues. Everyone must surely recognize that there is a lifetime worth of difference between 'family planning' and baby riddance. As the German Protestant theologian Helmut Thielicke said, 'Once impregnation has taken place it is no longer a question of whether the persons concerned have the responsibility for possible parenthood; they have already become parents.' If the parents exercise the privilege of sexual intercourse when there is a possibility pregnancy will occur, then they must likewise accept the responsibility for any pregnancy which may ensue from it.

"The argument that 'a woman has the right to control her own body' may be correct, but it is not the issue at this point. Once she is pregnant, that fetus is entirely separate, distinct, and unique. It is not part of her body, but only dependent on her body for nutrition and a safe environment."

Controlling abortion, Dr. Grady feels, is absolutely necessary if Western free society is to endure. "When the German physicians subordinated their ethics to the plan of Hitler, they became as, Dr. Andrew C. Ivy stated at Nuremburg, '. . . servants of the state, healers on the one hand, respected murderers on the other.' It was this loss of principle by the medical profession which subsequently prompted the Geneva Doctor's Declaration of the World Health Organization which states: 'I will maintain the utmost respect for human life from the time of conception; even under threat I will not use my medical knowledge contrary to the laws of humanity.'

"The permissive appetite that now allows abortion on demand will never be satisfied. Liberalization of the abortion law is but the first step for many of those most vigorously proposing abortion. It begins with 'updating archaic abortion laws' or 'abortion reform,' followed by liberal abortion, abortion on demand at any stage, infanticide, and euthanasia. One Nobel Prize scientist has already suggested that newborn babies be given tests and a period of evaluation. Those who meet the standards are then given birth certificates. The others are destroyed and considered not legally born.

"No physician, no parent, no hospital group, no legislative assembly or government," Dr. Grady declares, "has the right to take innocent life. As one senator stated, back when the Florida senate was debating as to whether the decision to 'terminate a pregnancy' should be left up to doctors or to lawyers: 'I offer a third alternative—that it be left up to God, and the child be permitted to live.'"

DR. THOMAS C. MONROE, JR., OBSTETRICIAN AND GYNECOLOGIST

Dr. Monroe, a physician for 27 years, has delivered thousands of babies. He is alarmed and dismayed at the increase in abortions.

"We've always had abortions, but not by the millions. Before the

Supreme Court ruling, New York State had allowed abortion on demand for about two years. Thousands of women flocked to New York. Many respectable medical centers were turned into abortion mills. Many physicians, who had sworn to uphold life, either advocated abortion on demand in principle or began to perform abortions. Then came 'Black Monday,' January 22, 1973 when the whole country became like New York. From my viewpoint as a Bible-believing Christian, the clock of time counting the 'last days' took a quantum leap forward. Second Timothy 3:1-7, which describes the perilous times just before the coming of the Lord speaks of the absence of natural affection. Millions of women are now 'without natural affection' (v.3, KJV) for their unborn.

"Normally, a woman who becomes upset at learning she is pregnant, will by the third or fourth month and certainly when movement is felt, develop natural maternal feelings toward her offspring. She'll want to protect it at all costs. But these women are without that natural maternal affection and demand abortions. Two thirds say they never feel any qualms."

Dr. Monroe believes life begins when the fertilized egg becomes attached to the uterus. Thus he does not classify the IUD and the "morning after" pill as abortion agents.

"The egg doesn't receive nutrients from the mother," he explains, "until implanted in the prepared surface lining of the uterus. At this moment it establishes its need for something other than itself. To my mind, preventing that from occurring is only preventing fertilization.

"Psalm 139 states that we are formed in the mother's womb, the uterus. Conception occurs in the fallopian tube, but implantation is in the womb."

After implantation, Dr. Monroe is "unalterably opposed" to abortion as a means of contraception or for convenience. He can only approve abortion for certain therapeutic reasons.

"Childbirth can still be fairly hazardous for some women. I can recommend abortion for a woman with severe hypertensive, cardiovascular disease, or if giving birth might jeopardize a woman's health so that she couldn't raise the children she already has.

"I can also perform an abortion when testing reveals the newborn will be so severely defective as to not have human characteristics. A hydrocephalic fetus, for example, more commonly known as a 'water-head,' will suffer atrophy or deterioration of the brain. It also frequently requires a cesarean section delivery. An acephalic, a baby without a head, can live only a vegetable life. To my way of thinking, such pregnancies should be terminated.''

The rare Tay-Sachs disease is another affliction which Dr. Monroe believes calls for abortion. A Tay-Sachs child appears normal at birth but within a few months, motor weakness sets in. As the central nervous system further degenerates, paralysis, blindness, and convulsions follow.

''Such congenital defects and deformities can financially drain the parents. In the case of a hydrocephalic or acephalic, they will have no offspring to communicate with. A Tay-Sachs child will be with them only a very short time and can literally bankrupt the family. It is a sin, I believe, not to terminate such pregnancies.''

A Downs syndrome (mongoloid) child is not a candidate for abortion for Dr. Monroe. ''I cannot understand a Christian aborting such a child. Mongoloids can be very special. They seem to lack the capacity for prejudice, hate, jealousy, self-pity, and resentments. I've never known one that wasn't a blessing to a family.''

Whether Dr. Monroe thinks an abortion is called for or not, he is required by the ''informed consent'' law to explain the options open to the woman and her husband. ''Early in the pregnancy I will tell a woman who runs a greater risk for a fetal deformity such as a Down's syndrome, 'If you insist, I will do an amniocentesis and let you know at 14 to 16 weeks if you are carrying a mongoloid.' We will discuss it and if she is a Christian, I will also ask, 'What will you do when you know, get an abortion?' She always answers, 'Of course not.' I do not do the amniocentesis and she awaits God's plan.''

Neither does Dr. Monroe recommend abortion for an unwed mother. ''There are 11 couples waiting for every adoptable baby,'' he notes.

''I don't believe it's heroic for an unwed mother to keep her child and raise it as a bastard without a father. The real heroine is one who has the courage to have the baby and give it up for adoption.''

The Tennessee physician ''has been amazed at the lack of involvement of the Protestant church in the abortion problem. The church has said little and done almost nothing in fighting this horrible stain upon our country. I have asked several pastors about this. Their answer has been that they don't want to touch 'sensitive social issues' for fear of turning someone off and not getting the opportunity to present the Person of Jesus Christ. There seems to be a dichotomy of direction here, but I will leave the problem with these pastors and pray for the success of such movements as Right-to-Life and Pro-Life. I do wish, however, that those people would give obstetricians a fence to sit on in these difficult situations. There is a zone between *abortion on demand* and *no abortion for any reason.*''

Dr. Monroe strongly favors sex education in the church. ''The schools provide only worldly sex education, although they could provide ethical sex education if they would. The church can give Christian, biblical sex education. It would make a difference.

''After you come to know Christ, you need to know what the Bible says about sex, children, and the sacredness of life. If the Bible doesn't speak to a problem, then I think you have a choice. Most Christians, I find, don't know what is scriptural and they're left to do as they please.''

Why does Dr. Monroe feel this way? ''Experience. Observation. I have patients all the time who hear the Bible, read the Bible, but never relate Scripture to life situations.''

Dr. Monroe himself became a Christian only a few years ago. ''I was never an atheist, except for a short time in my youth. That was a complete failure. It takes a bit of stupidity to believe there is no Creator. I don't see how anyone who delivers babies can *not* believe in God, because of the way the baby is formed in the mother's womb and the way it develops until the personality is born. The baby is born with personality from his very first breath. You can tell that this kid is different from that kid. It doesn't take sensitivity, just someone who will be observant.

''I was very moral, very ethical; more so, it seemed, than many of my so-called Christian acquaintances. I thought myself a better husband, a better father. I didn't know anyone who was as good as I was at that time.

''I thought I had it made. My marriage was next to perfect. I had two wonderful children, both doing well in the finest schools. I had a good income, and had reached the pinnacle of my profession. But still I wasn't satisfied.

"My wife Helen would often wish that our children had the comfort of prayer she had known as a child. I'd say to her, 'Even if Jesus wasn't who they said He was, He was still historically the greatest moral Teacher who ever lived.' Notice I said, 'who they said He was.' I didn't read the Bible. I didn't know this was what Jesus had said. But we decided to take our children to church.

"We were bored, but nobody called us sinners. Then we were talked into going to hear Ben Haden at First Presbyterian in Chattanooga. One of my friends had told me about this church where the pastor welcomed the congregation and himself as a bunch of sinners. Ben spoke my language. We started going regularly. After about a year we joined the church. I came to be an intellectual Christian. I was convinced; logically I believed. It was the only thing that made sense in this mixed-up world.

"I began to pray as instructed. Nothing happened. I'd drift off to sleep, miserable. If this was the abundant Christian life, they could keep it.

"Then a problem came that I couldn't handle. I had to go to bed with a bad back. As I worried about what would happen to my materialistic world if I couldn't practice, I became depressed beyond belief.

"The following morning I had a difficult operation scheduled. With the pain in my back, I didn't see how I could handle it. But I dressed and said, 'Okay, I'll try it one more time.' I fell down to my knees, and I said, 'Lord, help me! I can't do it by myself!' I knew I had connected. I went into that operating room convinced that the Lord was going to give me stamina to stand up for that long case. In shortly over an hour I was through. It was a tremendous success. I knew I hadn't done that case at all. God had. My ego was deflated—gone. God had shown me His will being done, not mine.

"The following Sunday I had an even more important lesson. We were standing in church, singing the hymn, 'I Am Thine O, Lord,' The chorus goes, 'Draw me nearer, nearer, nearer, blessed Lord, to Thy precious bleeding side.' Then it hit me! He did it! He really did it. He died for me!

"Christ entered into my life that day and has controlled most of it most of the time since. I've known a peace within that I've never known before. Through an entirely different experience, Helen has come to know Jesus. She walks with Him each day.

"We still have the material things. But they aren't as important anymore. We've come to know One who gives us real joy and guidance in the tough decisions.

"One of the toughest decisions I always have is whether to terminate a pregnancy. No other problem in my practice of obstetrics requires as much prayer."

DR. CARL WENGER, GENERAL SURGEON

The Little Rock doctor is "absolutely opposed to abortions performed for socioeconomic reasons. That's what abortion on demand has come to be now," he believes.

"I have never taken the hard line that if the mother's life is in danger the fetus cannot be sacrificed. But this situation is very uncommon.

"Whether to save or abort a child with defects has been a real struggle for me. I have concluded, after much thought, that if the decision were mine to make, I would not perform an abortion under those circumstances. A deformed child can be a tremendous burden to a young family in our society. Yet from the Christian perspective, I know of many instances where marvelous love has been demonstrated to a child with physical or mental limitations.

"I know a woman who gave birth to a grossly deformed, completely dependent child. Her husband died about a year ago. She has one other child. The deformed child must be a real heartache to her, and at the same time a tremendous source of a comfort. A surgeon friend of mine and his wife in Memphis have a little girl with cerebral palsy. Their whole family is built around this little girl. It's a thing of beauty to watch their care for her, to see the love of the other siblings.

"We can't measure this kind of love. It takes a unique person to handle something of this nature. When allowed to be in control, God the Holy Spirit can make of it a great blessing. I'm personally convinced that physically and mentally limited children fall into the 'all things' of Romans 8:28. God can use these 'tragedies' to conform us to the likeness of His Son."

DR. ROGER VEITH, CHATTANOOGA NEUROSURGEON

"I think there are some instances when a couple should have an abortion for medical reasons. With certain diseases, such as severe diabetes, or when the mother's life is endangered, I could justify an abortion. I might accept an abortion if a panel of experts decided it was best for serious psychological reasons. But to have an abortion just because you are pregnant and the child is unwanted—that's certainly wrong. A child with a chance of being defective I would leave in the hands of God.

"When I was doing my surgical residency, my wife contracted German measles when pregnant with our third child. This was at Duke University Medical School, a very conservative institution, and very strict about abortions. Mickey was in her third month when the doctors recommended the abortion route. We said, 'No, we can't do that. This is God's child, not ours. We don't know what He has planned for this child, but it's not our decision. We'll have to run the risk, if you want to call it a risk.'

"So against the doctors' advice, we had our little boy. He's now 14, in good health, doing well in school, and is a real joy to our lives."

5

Genetic Engineering: Quest for the Ideal Man

"You're pregnant," the doctor told Joan Meredith. "Fill out these forms and have the nurse schedule your next checkup."

The first form asked for the usual health history, the second, a list of inherited diseases. Down's syndrome, cystic fibrosis, and Tay-Sachs she'd heard of, but what was hemophilia? *Something to do with the blood,* she guessed. A memory crossed her mind. *Mother's only brother died of uncontrollable bleeding when he was 11.*

"Could you get your uncle's health records?" the doctor asked.

"He died out in the country. I don't think they did an autopsy."

"Well, we'd better have you checked with a geneticist. Just as a precaution. Ask the nurse to make you an appointment at the university hospital."

"Do I have it?" a worried Joan pressed.

"Women carry the trait. Only males can get it. Then there's a fifty-fifty chance of being normal."

Joan decided not to worry her husband Harry until she'd had the test. It was positive. She was a carrier.

"What next?" she asked the genetic counselor.

"Keep your regular prenatal appointments. At about 16 weeks we'll do an amniocentesis. We'll put a needle into the baby's amniotic sac and withdraw some amniotic fluid. That'll tell us the sex. If it's a girl, you're home free, except that she may be a carrier."

"And if it's a boy?" Joan asked.

"We'll do another test to see if he's a hemophiliac. That's a very new procedure. Before, you couldn't have known for sure until birth."

She told Harry all the details and gave him a pamphlet from the genetics counselor. "I had a customer with a hemophiliac child," Harry finally said. "He and his wife were afraid to let him out of their sight. The least little injury could start a hemorrhage." He paused, seeing Joan's drawn face. "But let's don't get alarmed until you have the next test."

During the next few weeks Joan and Harry read everything they could find about hemophilia. The disease played no favorites. Queen Victoria had been a carrier, passing the trait on to her granddaughter Alexandra, wife of Czar Nicholas of Russia, who in turn gave it to her son. A mad monk named Rasputin had gained a bizarre hold over Nicholas and Alexandra by convincing them he could control their son's bleeding. In his preoccupation with the boy, Nicholas allowed the country to drift until it was too late to stop the Communist revolution. Now, over six decades later, there is still no cure. Twenty-five thousand American boys have had the disease.

Joan and Harry brushed up on genetics, the science of heredity, a subject they had hardly thought about since high school days. They noted that the union of sperm and egg produces a cell with two sets of 23 chromosomes, one set from each parent, which determine the baby's physical and mental characteristics.

Each chromosome, they learned, is sectioned into genes which contain the "blueprints" for future development. A mutation or change in a gene can alter the blueprint, often changing the whole life of an individual.

Every person, they learned, inherits two genes for a particular trait, one from each parent. Often one will overpower the other. The stronger one is *dominant* and the weaker *recessive*. "That's why I have my faher's brown eyes instead of my mother's blue eyes," Harry exclaimed.

They found that the man determines the sex of the child. His sperm can contain either an X or a Y chromosome while the woman's egg carries only an X. If the sperm that fertilized the egg has an X, the product will be two Xs and a girl. If a Y, the sequence is XY and a boy will develop.

The X and Y sex-linked chromosomes are sometimes defective and may produce such diseases as color blindness, hemophilia, and muscular dystrophy. Males almost always get these diseases because they have just one X chromosome. Females have two Xs and the harmful effect of genes on one X is usually subdued by dominant genes on their other X.

The time came for Joan's amniocentesis test. The fetal fluid showed an XY chromosomal pattern—a boy. At least he wouldn't be a carrier and he might be normal. In the next test, the new one, a few drops of blood were drawn from one of the baby's blood vessels on the placenta. The blood was then analyzed by radio-immunoassay techniques for the blood clotting substance known as Factor VIII. "There isn't enough of the factor to count," the Merediths were told. "Your boy is likely to be a hemophiliac. We're sorry."

They were given the options of abortion, or keeping the baby and expecting to pay around $20,000 a year for regular injections of Factor VIII. With that there were no guarantees that their boy would finish high school. Would he be retarded? "No," the geneticist said, "He'll be normal in every way except for the hemophilia."

They prayed and agonized. Why would God allow this to happen? Abortion would be the easy way out, but they couldn't do it. "I believe our son is already a real person," Joan said. "We couldn't kill him after he was born and we won't kill him now. I'll take a job and we'll manage somehow. We have to believe God has a purpose."

Their son was born with golden hair and blue eyes, just like his father, and normally healthy. Before leaving the hospital, Joan was sterilized.

Defective Genes

It's understandable if Joan Meredith and thousands of other genetic disease carriers—both male and female—feel imperfect. Actually, every person has some defective genes. Ordinarily these bad genes are recessive, with their effects blocked by normal dominant genes. But when people with the same abnormal genes marry, thereby doubling the power of the bad genes, their chances of bearing a diseased child increase greatly. In some instances, the odds can jump from 1 to 25 to 1 in 4.

Statistical probabilities of genetic defects vary greatly. The chance of having a cyclops child, with one eye in the middle of the forehead, is 1 in 40,000. For Down's syndrome or mongolism, the odds increase with the mother's age—1 in 2,000 for women over 30; 1 in 100 for mothers past 35.

Some 2,500 known genetic human abnormalities can now be identified. About 100 of these can be discovered through genetic testing before birth. Others, while not recognizable to the naked eye, can be diagnosed by simple tests in the hospital nursery. Some abnormalities are little more than a nuisance—flat feet, for example. Some ravage the body and destroy the mind. Others kill within a short time after birth.

Down's syndrome can be detected by amniocentesis. Without the test, the mongoloid features are obvious at birth: broad short head, flat spadelike hands, and slanting eyes. Mental retardation is soon apparent also.

Tay-Sachs babies can also be identified by amniocentesis. Called the Jewish genetic disease (1 in every 3,600 Jewish births), Tay-Sachs results in blindness and painful seizures. Tay-Sachs babies usually do not live beyond their third birthday.

Huntington's chorea, unless discovered by testing, may not become known until age 35. Deficient in nerve impulses, victims jerk, twist, and shake uncontrollably. They are also prone to rages and paranoid delusions. Folk singer Woody Guthrie died from this disease after 15 years of suffering.

Many genetic defects can hasten heart disease, certain cancers, emphysema, and other dread diseases. Hypercholesterolemia, for example, is characterized by a deficiency in chemical agents that normally hold down cholesterol. Fatty deposits build up rapidly in the blood, clogging arteries. Unless precautions are taken, a victim may die of a heart attack in his 30s or even earlier.

The mental anguish resulting from known genetic diseases cannot be measured. The financial price tag is also enormous. The cost of treating Down's syndrome children alone is $1.7 billion a year in the U.S. and is rising.

Only the effects of hereditary afflictions can now be treated. Sufferers with cystic fibrosis, for example, must go to the hospital every few months and have excess mucus removed from their lungs. When their lungs collapse, they can live a while longer on a respirator.

A few genetic diseases can be treated more directly, if diagnosed in time. MMA (Methymalonic Acidemia), for example, is marked by lack of Vitamin B12 which causes mental and physical retardation. If it is detected in prenatal testing. The mother can be given superdoses of B12 which will penetrate the placenta barrier and be absorbed into the fetus. After birth the child will develop normally on a low-protein diet and daily doses of B12.

PKU (phenylketonuria) is caused by an inborn defect of protein metabolism. Left untreated, a PKU baby becomes moderately to severely retarded. The disease can be identified at birth from a pin prick of blood or a drop of urine. A special diet will usually check the retardation.

After having one PKU child, there is a one in four chance that a couple's next baby will have the same defect. Because the problem is treatable, a couple may wish to have more children.

Untreatable Diseases

Carriers of traits which can result in untreatable serious maladies face a much greater dilemma. A young woman who knows she is a carrier of a serious disease may choose not to marry. If she does, she may decide to be sterilized.

A married couple with one defective child will be fearful of taking a chance on another. They may opt for sterilization or artificial insemination if the husband's genes are the problem.

A couple with a known defective child on the way faces the hardest decision of all: abortion or the possibility or probability of bringing a seriously abnormal child into the world. Some couples with suspect genes may go ahead with the pregnancy and let amniocentesis be their guide. If the test results are positive, they have an abortion; if negative, their fears are allayed.

Christian Dilemma

There are no easy answers for Christians in these dilemmas. Some Christian physicians will abort a Tay-Sachs child, but not a mongoloid or hemophiliac.

Christians struggle with deep theological questions: "Why has God allowed this to happen to us? What purpose does He have? How can He be glorified?"

Generations before us were aware that certain diseases ran in families, but were not confronted with such complexities of choices. The questions which we now face are part of the price to be paid for increased knowledge and advances in medical science. Since we know more and can do more, we are confronted with a complicated stewardship. We look in vain for quick, easy answers.

The Bible has little to say about heredity. First Chronicles 20:6 tells of a Philistine warrior, the "son of a giant," with 12 fingers and 12 toes. Scripture speaks of "sons of the prophets" and "children of wickedness," but only in a moral and spiritual context. The chosen people were forbidden to intermarry with Canaanites, but this was apparently because of their neighbors' moral degeneracy and hostility to God, and not their genetic abnormalities.

We read in the Bible that the sins of the fathers were "visited" upon the children. These were moral transgressions. It was known then, for example, that venereal disease could affect one's children. This principle was incorrectly applied by many ancients to include *all* disease evident at birth. Jesus exposed this error. Of a man blind from birth, He said, "It was neither that this man sinned, nor his parents" (John 9:3).

From a theological perspective, defective genes are a part of the fallen creation. There is evidence today that at least some genetic problems have resulted from transgression of God's laws. Sickle-cell anemia is an example. The genetic mutation that causes the disease was for some black people a life-saving protection against malaria in the African environment of their forefathers, although others did die from anemia. When blacks were enslaved and brought to new climates in America, the sickle cells became more destructive.

Because of man's collective and individual disobedience the "whole creation groans and suffers" (Rom. 8:22). Is the fact that 99 percent of all genetic mutations are bad a part of this groaning? Some geneticists today believe that the human gene pool was cleaner in earlier times. If so, this may explain human longevity before the Flood.

More to the point, we can receive moral guidance from biblical principles in making the rough decisions demanded in modern genetics. Christian love is other-directed. Love will defend and protect fetal life, even at sacrifice to one's self. But love will not be reckless or irresponsible in bringing children with severe genetic diseases into the world. Love will think of those who must bear the expense of supporting these children. Love will find alternatives to the natural desire for parenthood, where danger is involved, perhaps in helping deprived children already born. Love, furthermore, works to alleviate human suffering and supports all worthwhile healing ministries, including ethical testing and research.

The critical test for genetic disease is now amniocentesis. It is 99.3 percent accurate, but is still controversial. Christian doctors have mixed feelings. "The whole system" (genetic prenatal testing), says Dr. C. Everett Koop, "is to find out if there is something wrong with the fetus. And if the fetus is defective some parents will decide to abort it. Since I take a high view of life, I see amniocentesis as a 'search and destroy' mission" (*Christianity Today,* December 15, 1978, pp. 340-1).

Parents are more apt to abort if they know something is seriously wrong with their child. Dr. John Fletcher, cochairman of the Institute of Society, Ethics, and the Life Sciences Study Group on Genetic Screening and Counseling, studied 25 couples of varied social, ethnic, and religious backgrounds who came for genetic counseling. All who were told that their children were defective chose abortion and then were sterilized.

Genetic counselors defend amniocentesis. Dr. Sara C. Finley of the University of Alabama asks critics to look at the testing another way:

"Many women with histories of genetic disease would be afraid to have a baby *without* amniocentesis" (*McCall's*, March 1979, as condensed in *Reader's Digest*, June, 1979, p. 112).

Genetic Roots

Genetic counseling is largely a phenomenon of the 1970s and is growing rapidly. Still only a small fraction of the estimated five million Americans with serious genetic problems are ever tested. Many couples marry without ever exploring their genetic roots. The result is that thousands of abnormalities in babies come as a complete shock to parents.

- Should applicants for a marriage license be required to present a genetic history?
- Should those with "suspect" heredities submit to genetic testing?
- Should known carriers of certain diseases be forbidden to marry?
- Should prenatal and postpartum (following childbirth) testing be mandatory? (The test for PKU, for example, costs about a dollar and could prevent a lifetime of retardation.)
- Should retarded and insane persons be sterilized?
- Should a retarded woman who gets pregnant be given an abortion against her wishes?
- Should genetic profiles be required for job applicants?
- Should insurance companies rate policyholders on the basis of their genes?
- Should the federal government have on file genetic records for national health planning?

Christian young people are bombarded with these questions in public high schools and colleges. Influenced by humanistic teachers, many students find such goals reasonable, even necessary. But there are other factors to consider: The freedom and value of the individual, the danger of control by elitist politicians and intellectuals, the potential of grading population by desirables and undesirables, and the possibility of regarding certain persons as subhuman.

The misapplication of genetics in modern history should trouble anyone. About a century ago Francis Galton, the "father of modern eugenics" and a cousin of evolutionist Charles Darwin, set out to eliminate the unfit from British society. He believed that curvature of the spine, club feet, and high-arched palate in the mouth were marks of criminality that could be passed from parent to child. Drunkenness and epilepsy were also signs of degeneration. Once "bad seed" was evident in a family, he said, the tainted should be kept from breeding.

Galton asked for laws to prevent reproduction by epileptics, feeble-minded, convicted criminals, and paupers. He favored giving certificates of genetic merit to "healthy" young men and women. Galton's program attracted support from many influential atheists and agnostics. Playwright George Bernard Shaw proclaimed that it was the only "religion that can save our civilization from the fate that has overtaken all previous civilizations" (*Pre-Meditated Man*, p. 99).

Galton's ideas caught fire in the United States; before the Civil War many southern slave owners had practiced selective breeding. White racists mobs castrated blacks suspected of raping white women. Mental institutions in both North and South sterilized hundreds of patients judged "unfit for reproduction." In a Kansas home for boys, 44 young men were castrated (*Pre-Meditated Man*, p. 99).

In 1907 the Indiana Legislature ordered sterilization of idiots, imbeciles, and the feebleminded. Virginia defense lawyers took a young feebleminded woman's case to the U.S. Supreme Court on grounds that the state had denied her equal protection of the law under the Fourteenth Amendment. The court ruled against her. "Three generations of imbeciles are enough," declared Chief Justice Oliver Wendell Holmes.

Public revulsion finally turned back the tide. In 1939, while the world slept, Hitler ordered the extermination of mental defectives, and incurables. Hospital staffs made out death lists. In some places, nurses and attendants put on the list everyone whom they disliked. More than 275,000 died before the Jewish Holocaust began.

Twenty years after the end of World War II, Dr. Patricia Jacobs reported from Scotland a linkage between violent behavior and the chromosomal sex abnormality XYY. Disclosure that Richard Speck, the Chicago mass murderer of nine nurses, was an XYY gave wide publicity to Dr. Jacobs' study. Other scientists developed a method to screen masses of newborns as well as adults with criminal records for the abnormality. Hope spread that criminality might be checked in a generation. Just before the testing was to get under way, other studies were revealed that did not support Dr. Jacobs' conclusions. Businessmen, factory workers, and even clergy had been found to have the XYY aberration.

A crusade to stamp out sickle-cell anemia in blacks was initiated by civil rights leaders in the late 1960s. Articles and TV documentaries vividly described how the disease caused oxygen-starved red blood cells to clump and clog blood vessels, resulting in painful swelling of the joints, damaged kidneys, and lowered resistance to infection.

Eight percent of all blacks were known to be carriers of "the blood trait that threatens to cripple or kill" (a popular quote). The difference between carrying the trait and having the disease became blurred. Civil rights leaders demanded free screening clinics. Some states made testing mandatory.

Suddenly blacks were faced with a new discrimination in employment. Airlines, for example, refused to hire blacks for flying duties for fear that lowering of oxygen supply could cause the disease. "Are you a carrier of sickle-cell anemia?" became a regular question in many job interviews. Some life insurance companies raised their rates for known carriers.

The National Academy of Science's Research Council became alarmed and hurriedly reported that the sickle-cell menace had been greatly exaggerated. There was no scientific warrant for limiting the employment of black carriers. Only a scant few would ever get the disease. One could have the trait and still be in good health.

The XYY and sickle-cell anemia fiascoes illustrate how good intentions can lead to harmful results. Governments must use extreme caution in passing laws which restrict the individual freedoms of genetically defective people.

Genetic Construction

The battles over genetic research, testing, and treatments are just beginning. The newest frontier in experimentation, genetic transplants, is already posing mind-boggling dilemmas.

Some scientists foresee a new, genetically perfect humanity. When the environment is free from pollutants and world peace is assured, Ideal Man will have an Ideal Kingdom, they say.

A few are even talking of human immortality. They think cells could be extracted at a young age and frozen, then injected at intervals to rejuvenate the body.

To understand this new frontier in genetics, let us look more closely inside the human cell. The 46 chromosomes in each cell contain thousands of genes and the genes hold miles and miles of twisted, ladder-like, thinner-than-gossamer strands of DNA (deoxyribonucleic acid). DNA is the blueprint of life, drawn up by the Creator, the Master Architect.

The rungs on a DNA ladder are built from four chemical molecules—adenine, guanine, cytosine, and thymine coded A, G, C, T. Each rung has two of these chemicals, joined in the middle. Since there are thousands of rungs in a single cell, the possible combinations of chemicals are staggering.

When the mother cell divides, the gene divides, and the DNA ladder divides. Each new half-ladder builds a new opposite half just like the one that had split off from it. This means that each new cell has the same blueprint as the first, continuing through the trillions of cells in a complete body.

The DNA blueprint for a specific protein is picked up by another nucleic acid, called messenger RNA (ribonucleic acid). Acting like a general contractor, messenger RNA makes out a list of "building materials" (amino acids) needed to make the protein. Another substance, transfer RNA, takes the list and floats out into the cell to gather the materials and bring them back to messenger RNA for assembly. Chemical "subcontractors" then begin building the body.

Genetic defects happen when the blueprint is flawed by an error in the DNA code—a "misspelled word" or "jumbled paragraph." Unless corrected, the flaws keep repeating as the cells divide. Human tissues then become like letters from an automatic typewriter which was programmed in error.

Scientists already know the code of life, the chemical building materials, and are rapidly learning "construction" combinations. By genetic engineering, they hope to replace defective building materials with perfect products brought in from outside the cell. This is no pipe dream or science fiction fantasy. As Dr. James Watson, the codiscoverer of the

DNA ladder told a congressional science subcommittee in 1972: "The code of life has been cracked and genetic engineering is on its way. . . . Under the magic wand of biology man is now becoming quite different from what he was. Great leaps have been taken in recent years. Scientists can now:

- Manufacture artificial genes in the lab as exact duplicates of genes found in some bacterium.
- Use a special enzyme as a chemical scalpel for dissecting delicate DNA into workable pieces.
- Transfer genes from one species of bacterium to another. Researchers are regularly transplanting genes from rabbits, fruit flies, frogs, and other living things into Escherichia coli, a well-known bacteria found in the intestines of humans and animals.
- Fuse bits of DNA from different organisms into a new package of heredity called recombinant DNA and introduce this into bacteria. As the bacteria grows, each new cell contains the recombinant DNA.
- Inject insulin-producing cells into diabetic rats. Experiments have shown that the rats' blood sugar quickly drops to normal levels. Within three to five years this may be possible for human diabetics.
- Treat some cancers with interferon, a hormonelike protein produced in the cells of some animals. Extraction of interferon from cells is extremely expensive; a millionth of an ounce costs around $1,500. Scientists are now trying to isolate the gene that orders interferon production in the cell. Once that is done, recombinant DNA can be used to insert it into a bacterium which will then multiply and produce large quantities of interferon.

The possibilities of transplanting and combining heredities in agriculture and animal husbandry are staggering. DNA from plants that possess nitrogen-processing abilities might be transferred to plants that do not, thus saving enormous amounts of fertilizer. DNA from fruits that do not freeze in cold weather might be spliced into genes of fruits that are not frost-resistant. Oranges might be grown in Indiana. Among animals, cows might be given the longer life span of elephants.

The potential for humans is even more mind-boggling. Genetic defects might be corrected at their source. Genetic engineers might sharpen senses and increase the physical stamina of limbs and organs.

Ideal Man would have supervision, superhearing, and would be able to run a one-minute mile.

Genetic Cautions

But there are rumblings and fears. Fears that DNA-juggling, like nuclear fission, might become more of a curse than a blessing. Fears that zealous scientists might inadvertently let a "doomsday bug" lose in the world which could spread genocidal strains of a new disease. Such worries prompted alarmed American scientists to call a moratorium on all recombinant DNA research until safety guidelines could be drawn up. But no one believes that guidelines, even if followed by all researchers, are foolproof. There are too many unknowns out ahead.

- Who will be wise enough to decide which traits are worth keeping and which should be "corrected"?
- Could a mad dictator reshape a population to his liking?
- What will genetic engineering do to human nature?
- Can gene splicing eradicate the sin nature?
- Who will bear responsibility for choices?
- Can people blame their misfortunes on genetic engineers?

After listing six pressures upon society, Francis Schaeffer said, "There is a seventh pressure which is the greatest yet. Especially in Europe scientists are wrestling with this. It is often called the biological bomb, a bomb much greater than the hydrogen bomb. I am not being spectacular: Within 20 years we will be able to make the kind of babies we want to make. The genetic engineers have made most of the basic breakthroughs on this.

"Modern man has no moral imperative for what he *should* do, and consequently he is left only with what he *can* do. And he is doing what he can do even though he stands in terror. And the biggest terror of all is: Who is going to make the babies? Who is going to know what kind of babies we need to make? Who is going to shape the human race?" (*The Church at the End of the 20th Century*, InterVarsity Press, 1976, pp. 87-88)

Professor Paul Ramsey of Princeton opposes any experiment in genetic engineering, such as introducing a virus to alter a defective gene, unless it is known that no hazards will be involved. The Princeton scholar holds that no parent has a right to give proxy consent for a child born or unborn to a procedure intended primarily for research and not planned for the good of the patient.

Norman Anderson, recently retired as professor of Oriental Laws and director of the Institute of Advanced Legal Studies at the University of London and known as a "theologian among lawyers," states his concern in his recent book *Issues of Life and Death*. "Nature is not inviolable, for nature itself has been affected by cosmic sin. Nor is there anything wrong with man acting as a "creative manipulator," provided that he always remembers that he is exercising only a delegated authority, that he is himself prone to both sin and error, and that he must do his utmost never to act contrary to the essence or implications of the revealed will of the Creator Himself—judged, *inter alia,* in terms of the reverence due to man made in the image of God, of the family structure in which he has been placed, and of his duty of service to the human race as a whole" (InterVarsity Press, p. 57).

Henry Stob is Professor Emeritus of Philosophical and Moral Theology at Calvin Theological Seminary, Grand Rapids, Michigan, and founder and editor of *The Reformed Journal*. He writes, "A conviction governing a great deal of the scientific concern with man is that man is not a finished product of creation but is an unfinished, malleable and openended something, which, having been produced by Mother Nature, is being moved by evolutionary forces into a promising future. It is this conviction which justifies for many scientists the various forms of genetic engineering. Biomedical science, in this context, is not concerned, as it was in the past, simply to support or heal; it is concerned to program and direct, and in this way to be as creative as nature itself.

"A Christian should, I think, not ignore the dynamic aspects of human existence, but neither should he lose sight of the static structures which set limits to man's nature and within which the elements of potentiality are confined. Because man is divinely structured I find it hazardous, if not impious, to tamper with the genetic core. To tamper with the genes seems to me to outrun God into an unknown future and to exercise an elective discrimination mere men do not possess" (*Ethical Reflections,* Eerdmans, pp. 220-222).

6

Christian Perspectives on Genetic Engineering: Quest for the Ideal Man

DR. LANE P. LESTER, GENETICIST

"What lies ahead for the human species?" Dr. Lester asks rhetorically. "Assuming," he says, "that we don't wipe ourselves out with a nuclear holocaust or pollution. Or that God doesn't call a halt to time.

"Let's divide the question into what can *nature* do and what can *humans* do?

"Nature changes us by heredity and by mutations. There's nothing very fancy about heredity. It's simply the process that results in children looking something like their parents, but not exactly like either one. Through this process we receive half of our heredity from father and half from mother. Each generation is different from the previous generation.

"How much change is possible through inheritance? Quite a lot. Scientific breeding can produce many variations in plants and animals. No new varieties are ever bred. Change is within a species. A cat remains a cat, a fowl a fowl, and so on.

"Mutations, which cause the second kind of change, are genetic mistakes, errors that occur in passing the heredity from one generation to the next. How much change is possible through mutations? Consider the fruit fly, which geneticists have been experimenting with for almost 70 years. Some 3,000 mutations have been discovered in this one species.

"Mutations are almost always harmful—99.9 percent, some scientists say—and at best, are neutral in their effects. Not much hope here for improving the human race.

"Now if mutations are as bad as I've made them out to be, and they are, you may wonder why hasn't life been mutated right out of existence. A process called natural selection protects species against harmful mutations by eliminating or keeping down the number of life forms in which harmful mutations occur. Natural selection also has a positive role. It helps a species to adapt to its environment.

"We don't know nearly as much about human genetics as we do about fruit flies. We can't use the same experimental techniques. For one thing, humans don't reproduce as fast as fruit flies. You have to wait years and years to see what happens. It becomes very difficult to separate environment from genetics. It's also hard to make nice, pat statements about such abstracts as intelligence.

"But we do know that heredity, mutations, and natural selection all affect humans.

"What about genetic engineering? Since the Son of God Himself made healing a major part of His ministry, I think He wants us to do all we can about the thousands of defective children born every year. But many genetic engineers want to control and manipulate the processes of heredity to their designs, getting rid of or correcting all the mutants. That's a pretty big order.

"Some propose to do this by abortion, sterilization, and euthanasia of the unfit. That was basically Hitler's program, although I don't mean to imply that today's genetic engineers are Nazis. The ones I've met are decent, sincere people who want to help humanity. Most, however, don't see a spiritual dimension to man. They think man must be in control of his own destiny.

"Let's look at positive genetic engineering. The idea is to replace or subdue bad heredity with good. It is possible now to chop DNA up and package it in viruses, then use those viruses to transfer the controlled DNA into animal cells. This has fantastic implications for the future, but it is also fraught with problems.

"Take the effort to put insulin-making DNA into the cells of diabetics. A cure for diabetes and other diseases which may have connections to bad genes sounds wonderful. But this good result could increase the "pollution" in the human gene pool, since more persons with defective DNA would reproduce and pass their heredity problems to offspring. A second concern is that some germ might escape a lab and infect the rest of us. It could wipe out the human race.

"In general, I think we can trust scientists to correctly report the facts. What matters, however, is the standard and philosophy under which scientists work. Many believe that man is just an evolved animal, responsible only to himself. For them, anything possible is permissible.

"Humans have dignity because they have spiritual natures. Human engineering to correct mental and physical defects can be very beneficial, but unless those who receive this benefit also receive God's cure for their sin, it will be like putting cosmetics on a cancer."

DR. V. ELVING ANDERSON, HUMAN GENETICIST

Besides teaching and researching, Dr. Anderson is a genetic counselor and acting director of the Dight Institute of Human Genetics.

"I talk with families who are, or think they may be, genetic risks. To illustrate: Here's a family where the husband is 41 and the wife 40; they have four children, one of whom died in infancy. At their ages they are wondering, 'Can we have another child?' I must tell them that their chances of having a Down's syndrome baby are three to five percent, and that a test can be made during pregnancy which will indicate what kind of defect, if any, can be predicted. I am not making the decision for them. I am just giving them the facts and the alternatives. They will then decide. It's been my experience that most of those who have the test and learn that they have a Down's syndrome fetus will terminate the pregnancy."

Dr. Anderson reports that genetic testing is becoming safer and more accurate. "The doctor uses ultrasound prior to amniocentesis to locate the placenta and ensure that the needle will be inserted where it will be of least harm. Ultrasound can be used to diagnose dwarfism, because the sound waves make it possible to visualize the fetus and determine the relative proportions of the arms and legs. It can also pick up heart sounds and diagnose a heart defect in the fetus.

"One of the newest techniques is fetoscopy. The physician inserts a larger needle than the one used in amniocentesis, one that uses fiber optics to transmit light and convey a picture. You can visualize the fetus. You can look at blood vessels on the surface of the placenta, insert a needle and withdraw blood from the fetus for examination.

"A whole range of testing techniques is now being introduced. Unfortunately, for the most part, these do not detect conditions for which positive intervention is possible. The percentage of cases that can be helped is still very small. In principle, it will always be possible to diagnose more problems than can be treated.

"Sometimes high levels of vitamins can be administered that will help the fetus without hurting the mother. When a baby's defective enzymes cannot handle the normal food intake, a special diet after birth will help. One can try to go a step further by giving good enzymes, but enzymes are more difficult to administer than hormones (which naturally circulate in the blood stream and have an effect on cell surfaces). Most enzymes in the blood are broken down very rapidly. Furthermore, the enzymes have to get inside a cell, in most cases, to be effective. So there are experiments to stabilize enzymes by modifying some part of their structure adding part of a molecule to make them acceptable to specific organs of the body. The idea is to put an address label, so to speak, on enzymes, so they will be picked up by the liver, if that's where they are needed."

Dr. Anderson estimates there are about 40 rare genetic traits which lead to a greater risk of developing some cancers. "They do not always lead to cancers," he stresses, "but they may, given the susceptibility and certain environmental factors. For example, some individuals have a genetic tendency for skin changes. When exposed to sunlight they develop unusually heavy freckling. Some of these spots can develop into skin cancers.

"We know there are some viruses that will cause cancers in experimental animals. The difference between a particular cancer-causing virus, and a virus that does not, is a single gene. There's so much we don't know about the connection between heredity and environment. We think environmental conditions may set things off that are in the body because of genetic defects. But we usually can't be sure. It is known that asbestos contributes to cancer. But why do some asbestos workers get cancer and others do not? It may be that the difference is in their genes.

"Presently I am doing genetic studies of epilepsy. We can list about 120 rare genetic conditions that lead to an increase in seizures. But all together, these genetic conditions account for only a very small fraction of the cases.

"Take the specific case of febrile convulsions in children. These children will have an infection and a high fever before suffering seizures. When this happens, we find the occurrence among siblings to be about ten percent as compared with about two percent in the general population. There may be a genetic cause for the likelihood that the brain will respond."

Dr. Anderson is sensitive to fears that "stress on genetic causes for human problems may take attention away from social factors which may also relate to the same problems. People think genetics can give us a quick fix; then we don't have to be concerned about the social situation of welfare recipients. Or we might blame aggression on an extra chromosome instead of looking for social pressures that lead to it. It is likely that there are genes which can help contribute to aggressive tendencies. But simply to say a single gene predisposes one to violence is absurd."

Dr. Anderson does not believe that genetics can fully define human nature. One has to guard against the thought that explanation of human nature at one level precludes explanation at another level. We can talk about biological explanation of human nature while realizing that when we have done our best, this is still not the heart and core of the totality of the individual. One can look at an individual as a spiritual being, and as a psychological, social, and biological being, and all these viewpoints can be compatible.

"If it were not for the Scriptures we could not deduce the view of God to whom we are responsible. That dimension comes to us from revelation. Knowing and learning more about genetics does not detract from that view, or from one's responsibility to God.

"Some have argued that there is a sense in which we are not totally free in our actions. I can't prove this. But I do know that the Scriptures treat us as having the ability to respond to God and being responsible for our responses. We need to consider these various ways of looking at the human race as complementary to each other.

"Those who reject belief in God ponder the human tendency to want ultimate explanations. Some scientists say humans shouldn't have these yearnings. This is kind of an indirect testimony to a dimension beyond biology, psychology, and sociology.

"There is a sense," Dr. Anderson admits, "in which our prior commitments influence the way we interpret the evidence. A growing knowledge of the complexities of life can lead to a greater reverence, for those of us who already believe in God as Creator and Sustainer. Our world view or philosophy of life becomes important to the way we understand these things."

Dr. Anderson finds no reason why Christian young people should be not interested in scientific research. "Sometimes, there is the impression that doctors serve God only when they directly minister to human suffering. This underestimates the possibilities of honoring God by scientific research. After all, God did command in Genesis that we should control and subdue. There are strategic areas of research and studies related to ethics which Christians need to explore."

DR. ROBERT L. HERRMANN, PROFESSOR BIOCHEMISTRY

As chairman of the Ethics Committee of the Christian Medical Society and a professor at a Christian medical school, Dr. Herrmann is especially concerned about ethics in science, particularly genetics.

"As amniocentesis gives us data on a baby before birth, it is opening a Pandora's Box for a whole new set of questions. We can know if the child is suffering from dwarfism, Down's syndrome, or some other defect. We have to decide at 16 or 17 weeks of pregnancy whether we want the child. Really, the more of this type of technology we achieve, the more choices are thrust upon us. Now that may be all right at the individual level, but suppose we were to say, 'God has given us this mongoloid child and we intend to keep it.' It's conceivable that 10 or 20 years from now a U.S. government agency may say, 'You cannot have that child. We will not support it in an institution.' And the government, in a cost-effective sense, has a right to say that it can't handle any more mongoloids.

"The questions get larger when we get into DNA transferral. It's easy for molecular biologists to feel with the great Jacques Monod that genetics is the gateway to all essential knowledge needed to guide the future of man.

"A considerable number of persons, including some scientists, have mixed feelings. An early fear was that harmful microbes, those carrying tumor-inducing genes in particular, might be loosed in the environment. A study committee from the National Academy of Sciences saw enough validity in this possibility to ask for a temporary moratorium in 1974. The following year about 140 scientists met in California and agreed on some general guidelines. A few lawyers were there to present possible liabilities.

"The work goes on to correct genetic defects at the gene level. Fears are still being expressed. Some, such as Dr. Robert Sinsheimer of Cal Tech, still think safety is a major problem. I tend to lean a little bit this way, but I'm not greatly alarmed. So far as I know, researchers are scrupulous in using microbes that can't live outside the laboratory. I don't think we need fear an *Andromeda Strain* escaping, which could infect the population. But I feel this kind of research should be done in a spirit of prayer and reverence. As Francis Bacon urged, 'We should approach with humility and veneration to unravel the volume of Creation'.

"I am concerned about experiments on humans. I wonder if we have the right to risk lives for the sake of a few more years of improved life in terms of a gene that is missing or is not completely functional. I've suggested to some colleagues that the experiments be done with human cells in culture instead of in a living body."

Dr. Herrmann sees a crisis in ethics in today's scientific community. He recalls the concern expressed by one of the world's outstanding biologists at an American Scientific Conference on Human Engineering at Wheaton College. "Our guest speaker confided that he was alone at his institution in his interest and burden for bioethics. He was very pleased to be in an environment where people were really looking at the issues and asking whether we should do these things and how we should do them. He was interested in our philosophical base and in our thought processes as Christians.

"According to one study, a very small percentage of scientists have any interest at all in ethics. These are the people who are making the tools for tomorrow's scientific technology. They have no philosophical framework for what they believe. Many, like Jacques Monod, admit they have no objective basis, no principles to live by. Monod concedes that today's scientists have been brought up beholden to Judeo-Christian principles. Even their humanism is derived from the basic value that man was created in the image of God. Monod considers these principles inadequate and wants to throw them away. He's an atheist, but he admits he has nothing else. Many scientists will not even face this lack.

"Another concern is that scientific research today is becoming more beholden to government for financing. My friend Walter Hearn, a biochemist, went through a moral struggle over acceptance of several grants for his research at a university. In the process of acceptance, he says that you accept the manipulation of your ideas and your goals. You gradually become subservient to the granting agency. Walter later resigned from the school.

"This isn't totally different from the situation in Nazi Germany. Hitler's scientists were given some rationalization for their work. They were destroying certain people to improve humanity. The fact that it was possible there suggests that it could happen here.

"The point I'm making is that the political system can control the scientists of a country. In the Soviet Union, for example, a botanist named Lasenko convinced Stalin back in the 30s that genetics was incompatible with the development of Communism. As a result, genetics was suppressed in Russia for about 25 years. That the Russians still haven't developed an effective agricultural system can be attributed to this policy."

The danger lies in the policies which scientists could follow, Dr. Herrmann emphasizes. "Science itself is not an enemy of faith. Modern science came out of a Christian culture. The early scientists believed the Creator was utterly trustworthy and His universe was ordered and rational. Einstein later echoed these convictions when he said that God 'is not arbitrary or malicious.' Einstein, of course, was not a Christian in the biblical sense. But he did see order and meaning in the universe, something which modern self-authenticating existentialism does not. 'It doesn't matter what you believe,' they say, 'so long as you believe it.' And, 'whatever turns you on is okay'.

"The holistic scientist, and the holistic theologian as well, recognize that there are many descriptions of reality. None are complete or exhaustive or exclusive. For example, the theologian might say, 'A rose is God's herald of summer'. The scientist might say, 'A rose is that part of the rose plant that bears the reproductive apparatus: the stamens, the pistil, the petals, and so forth'. Each is a valid description of a rose, but each says something quite different. We scientists must also see that we do not 'wrest from Nature her secrets' but rather we are *given* truth about creation by God with the expectation that we will act in responsible freedom."

Dr. Herrmann feels "very strongly" that Christians have the overarching, ultimate answers which the scientific world desperately needs. "I agree with Donald Mackay, the brain physiologist from England, who told our Wheaton conference, 'We can't leave well enough alone because things are not well.' The moral issue is not simply to say, 'We won't do that!' It might be immoral to do nothing. So we can't just walk away. There are people in need, and we've got to deal with them.

"To me, it is clear from Scripture that God has a heart for every man. As redemptive agents, we should not be secluded, but involved in the world. We should be finding our way into the decision-making roles in our society, and not be content just to be God's little flock."

7
Brain Research and Treatments of the Mentally Ill

An attractive piece of costume jewelry worn on the lapel? No, what appear to be tiny jewels are actually electric signal activators. Certain number sequences are tuned to electrodes in control centers of your brain. At the push of a tiny button you can change moods, alter sensations, stimulate memories, and shift perceptions. If you're angry with your boss and you see him approaching, you push 6824 for calmness. If it's Monday morning and you're feeling down in the dumps, you push 3312 for mild euphoria.

If this sounds wonderful, consider that your electronic stimulator and everyone else's is at the command of master controllers manning higher voltage stimulators that can overrule signals of the peasantry. At their leader's request, they can manipulate moods and feelings in areas of the population as desired, by states or counties, age groupings, and vocational classifications. By pushing the right buttons, they can cause farmers in Iowa to work harder; cool the anger of rebellious students at

Harvard; and calm the anxiety of auto assembly-line workers in Detroit who are fearful of losing their jobs because of automation. In sum, the leader, through his controllers, can manage the economy, prevent riots, lower crimes of passion where the murder and rape rates have been up, and restore emotional tranquility where a flood threatens.

Science fiction? Impossible? Not in the minds of some brain researchers who say this scenario could become reality by the year 2,000, under a sophisticated totalitarian dictatorship.

Look at what has already happened. In 1966 Dr. Jose Delgado, a Yale Medical School professor, jumped into an arena to confront an angry bull, carrying only a cape and a signal transmitter. He made a few passes with the cape and the bull charged. Then he pushed a button on the transmitter and the threatening bull slammed to a halt in its tracks.

The explanation: Several days before Delgado had implanted, in the center of the bull's brain, electrodes which inhibit aggression. When he signaled, the bull instantly became docile.

Hundreds of less spectacular experiments have been performed on other animals. Cats, dogs, and monkeys have been "commanded" to walk, run, stand still, attack, and become sexually aroused.

Electrodes have also been implanted in human brains. Scientists at Tulane University's School of Medicine placed 14 electrodes in the brain of a 28-year-old man who kept falling asleep while at work. They gave him a transistorized stimulator to wear on his belt. When he felt himself dozing off, he pressed a button and instantly became fully awake. Pressing other buttons brought different reactions.

Another subject was a 20-year-old woman confined to a hospital for the criminally insane. She frequently flew into violent rages and had to be kept under close watch. A university scientist attached an electrode to her brain and found he could trigger outbursts with a remote signal transmitter. By pinpointing the troubled area, he hoped to devise a treatment to bring the rages under control.

Electrical stimulation of the brain (ESB) is still largely in the experimental stage. The procedure is fairly simple for a trained neurosurgeon. Tiny holes are drilled through the skull at carefully selected places, and fine wires with electrode tips inserted into the brain. The type of response depends on where the electrodes are implanted. Dr. Delgado reports that in humans ESB has produced memories, fears of unknown dangers, friendliness, aggression, and changes in emotions and thinking processes.

Delgado scoffs at any possibility of governmental control through ESB. First, he says, implanting everyone's brain with electrodes will never be practical. Second, no two brains are exactly alike. Third, stimulating the same brain area in different individuals doesn't produce the same response. He sees the research as totally benevolent and notes that subjects suffering depression, intractable pain, epilepsy, anxiety, and involuntary movements have been helped.

ECT and Psychosurgery

Two better-known treatments of brain and mind disorders are electro-convulsive therapy (ECT), also called electric shock treatments, and psychosurgery. Publicity generated by a spate of nightmarish books and the movie, *One Flew Over the Cuckoo's Nest,* has magnified the number and effects of these procedures out of proportion with reality. Horrendous stories from dissidents released from Soviet mental hospitals have heightened public antipathy against such practices. The Soviet use of psychiatry and associated surgery as a political tool against dissenters was condemned by the World Psychiatric Association in 1977.

Despite fears engendered in popular science fiction and other literature, ECT is used with extreme reluctance and under close supervision. Trained personnel can easily administer ECT with proper equipment. The patient is put in a stupor with medication. Electrodes are taped to his temples and a 110-volt current shot into his brain for about 50 seconds. The shock may be repeated at intervals up to about a dozen times. The treatment is considered relatively safe, though amnesia and other complications sometimes occur. It usually lifts the depression enough for the psychiatrist to get at the root of the patient's problem. Ernest Hemingway, reportedly a manic-depressive, was given ECT treatments at the Mayo Clinic before his suicide. But some cannot be helped and one in a thousand die as a result of ECT. ECT is also administered as aversion therapy for behavioral modification of patients who cannot otherwise break a destructive habit. An alcoholic, for example, may be given a small shock each time a drink is set before him.

Psychosurgery conjures up an image of a mad scientist hovering over a helpless patient, grinning in fiendish delight at the prospect of cutting away a portion of the brain. There are undoubtedly a few mad psychiatrists (the profession leads all others in suicides) just as there are mad plumbers and carpenters. The psychosurgery—lobotomy—which provided this type of imagery for writers and film makers is an exaggerated hangover from the past which still haunts psychiatry. Also known as "ice-pick" surgery because of the type of instrument used, it involved cutting into the frontal lobe of the brain and severing certain connections. About 40,000 such operations were done in the 1940s. Until the 1950s it was the only way to treat some grave functional brain disorders. There was always risk involved. Many patients were helped dramatically, but some suffered loss of memory and interest in life, and a few died.

Psychosurgery today is much more precise and less dangerous. In a process called stereotaxis, the neurosurgeon drills a tiny hole in the skull and injects air or dye into ventricular open spaces in the brain. Then by X ray the doctor locates the diseased part of the brain by the distance it lies from a ventricle. The surgery is done by inserting a long needlelike device with an electrode tip. When the electrode reaches the target, the surgeon destroys the affected part by an electric current. This may relieve the symptoms of an otherwise incurable mental illness. However, mental illness does not always result from brain tissue which can be identified as physically diseased.

Only about 700 such operations are now being done each year in the United States. These are performed only when all else fails and under the most careful supervision. Under federal government rules, no patient can be operated on without his consent. Many psychiatrists say brain surgery should never be done on anyone for a behavioral disorder.

A neurosurgeon deals more often with more obvious physical problems in the brain, such as aneurysms, tumors, infections, and head injuries caused by accidents. CAT (computerized axial tomography) scanning and ultrasound help him pinpoint diseased areas. Microsurgery enables him to remove some tumors once thought untouchable. Radiation therapy, applied with high-energy devices, can sometimes destroy a malignant growth. No longer is brain cancer a certain ticket to death. At least 30 percent of such patients survive five years or longer.

Biochemical Drugs

ECT and psychosurgery have largely been made obsolete by biochemical drugs which work wonders never before dreamed possible. The biochemical revolution began with tranquilizers in the 1950s. Calming medication emptied mental hospitals by almost two thirds. But researchers were puzzled as to why the drugs worked on some patients and failed for others. Extensive research led to the discovery of 20 chemical neurotransmitters which ''jump'' messages at decision points between nerve cells. Further study convinced scientists that many physical and behavioral disorders are caused by imbalances among those brain chemicals. New drugs were developed to restore the natural order. Some dramatic results have been achieved.

Take, for example, Parkinson's disease, a nervous disorder with symptoms of muscle stiffness, trembling, stooped posture, rigidity in the face, and difficulties in walking, speaking, and writing. Researchers discovered that some patients suffered a deficiency in a neurotransmitter called dopamine. The drug L-Dopa was developed to correct the imbalance, bringing marvelous relief to many sufferers previously considered hopeless.

Another example is hyperkinesis which afflicts thousands of children. Victims have trouble with concentration, remembering, coordination of hands and eyes, and have a shortened attention span. They are often tagged in school as slow learners, even as retarded. Deficiencies of two crucial brain chemicals, noradrenalin and dopamine, were found in the brains of such children. Medication was produced that helps many, preventing them from developing serious psychological problems.

Severe depression has been linked to low levels of dopamine, noradrenalin, and a chemical compound called serotonin. Investigators found these chemicals could be destroyed by an enzyme known as monoamine oxidase (MAO). To prevent MAO's deadly work, biochemists produced a group of antidepressants called MAO inhibitors.

Serotonin has been connected to insomnia. It was already known that the body makes serotonin from a chemical called tryptophan, found in milk and some other foods. Experiments showed that tiny doses of tryptophan can put insomniacs to sleep.

Research into brain chemicals and the developments of additional drugs with more precise applications continue at a rapid pace. The field abounds with wide-eyed speculation and predictions that science may soon find an explanation of how Indian fakirs can walk over hot coals and not be burned, how acupuncture works, and why some soldiers lose limbs and feel little pain while others writhe in agony.

An Emory University scientist, Dr. Kalidas Nandy, is trying to develop a drug that will slow the destruction of brain cells now inherent in the aging process. He has pinpointed a cell-killing antibody which breaks through the "blood brain barrier system" at about the age of 25. As age increases, he says, the barrier further weakens, allowing more of the antibody to seep into the brain, dooming more brain cells. A stroke may damage the barrier to the extent that the antibody kills off large segments of the brain. If the manufacture of the antibody can be stopped, brain cells will survive longer, and the mind remain sharp, until a fatal disease comes along.

Behavior Modification

Such delving into the brain's chemical mechanisms brings only praise to medical researchers. But fears arise when scientists begin to talk of drugs that alter emotions, change feelings, modify behavior, and even change personality.

Are drugs with these capacities here? Consider the potency of eight general types.

● *Hallucinogens* are powerful mind expanders. A hundred micrograms of LSD, 1/175,000,000th of a man's body weight, can cause him to lose all control of time and space. Another major hallucinogen, mescaline, can produce similar psychological effects when taken in larger quantities.

● *Euphoriants* make a person so moronically optimistic that he loses touch with reality. Everything is "the best, the greatest."

● *Depressants* have the opposite effect of euphoriants, plunging a taker into morbid gloom where nothing is worth doing.

• *Cataplexogenics* keep the taker fully conscious, while his muscles are immobilized.

• *Disinhibitors* weaken or block controls in the brain that have kept behavior at a certain level. Alcohol is the most familiar disinhibitor.

• *Tranquilizers* reduce tension and nervousness.

• *Stimulants,* also called "mood elevators" and "psychic energizers," stimulate the arousal areas of the brain.

• *Opiates* (morphine, heroin, etc.) depress or deaden certain areas of the brain, stupefying a person to the degree and potency of narcotics ingested, shutting off troublesome sensations of the body.

These are only general types. Some can be purchased over the counter, some grown, some are bought illegally, and some are carefully controlled by prescription. Some have been used for thousands of years, but never before have such drugs been taken so widely, and never before has medical science had in its arsenal so many finely honed varieties of chemicals that affect the brain and nervous system.

Future Change

What of the future? Nuclear chemist Dr. Glenn T. Seaborg believes the next few decades may bring pharmaceuticals which change and maintain human personality at any desired level.

Already some scientists are talking of drugs to improve intelligence while other researchers are trying to transfer memories from one life to another.

Dr. James V. McConnell of the University of Michigan trained flatworms to react in a specific way to light. He cut up the trained worms and fed the bits to untrained worms. Then he tested the cannibals and found they responded to light the same way the trained worms had.

Dr. George Ungar of the Texas Medical Center shocked a rat each time it tried to enter a dark hole. When the rat was trained, he removed chemicals from the rodent's brain and isolated a chemical that he thought caused the rat to be afraid of the dark hole. He copied this chemical in the lab and injected samples into normal rats which habitually hid in dark places. These rats refused to enter the dark hole.

The most bizarre idea is brain transplants. A Russian claims to have transplanted the head of a dog to another canine body and kept the brain functioning for several days. Dr. Robert J. White, a neurosurgeon associated with Western Reserve University in Cleveland, and a team have transplanted 10 monkey heads and kept them alive a week. Dr. White thinks a human brain might be easier to transplant.

There is more serious talk of building a "cyborg"—an automated machine "man" which receives instructions from the biological "first man." This is not a clone but an extension and a magnification of normal man's functions. A cyborg might be used in space flight, for example. The idea is not so farfetched as it might seem when advances in mechanical arms and computers are considered. A *machine sapiens*, in which a human brain and nervous system are attached to an artificial body, is more fantastic.

Memory transfer, brain transplants, and cyborgs may be too far out, even impossible for humans. Electronic and drug instrumentation in brain therapy now confront us with profound questions which scientists are unable to answer. Dr. Wilder Penfield, a great Canadian neurosurgeon, notes that science throws no light on the nature of the spirit of man or God.

Nature of Man

● *What is man?* Is he only blood and flesh and bone with emotions, feelings, desires, fears, and inhibitions determined and regulated by chemicals in the brain?

● Or is he a "living being," as stated in Genesis 2:7, with mind and spirit, created by God in the Divine Image, and free and responsible?

● Is he also, because of the Fall, a sinner by nature and choice, yet with the capacity to respond to God personally through redemption offered in Christ?

● Or is sin only the result of chemical imbalances, flaws in evolution?

● Why is man here?

● Only to climb an evolutionary ladder, as he perfects his own species through biology?

● Or is he here as a steward of God's world, a servant of his fellows, a witness of God's majesty and power in creation and redemption?

- Where is man going?
- Are achievements during his biological life span and his physical posterity to be his only immortality?
- Is he ultimately, by his own genius, to extend his consciousness in other forms?
- Or is he destined, by his own choice, to spend eternity with God or separated from God?

The humanists' and Christians' answers are poles apart. There can be no middle ground.

As with genetic engineering, there is the question of control over the new brain therapies. There are, apparently, safeguards over ECT, psychosurgery, and brain experiments on humans. The U.S. Department of Health, Education, and Welfare will not provide federal funds to any institution which does not have a review board that passes on the ethical merits of each research project involving humans. But what of human engineering on a larger scale?

Two Fears

One evangelical authority speaking to these questions is Dr. Craig W. Ellison, chairman and professor of psychology and urban studies at Simpson College in San Francisco. "The motivation behind human engineering research is, for the most part, commendable," wrote Dr. Ellison in *Christianity Today*, January 19, 1979, p. 16. "The scientists want to alleviate suffering by the correction of genetic or behavioral defects, therapeutically control and rehabilitate those who are societally dangerous, and improve the overall functioning and future potential of the human race. . . . Few people would argue with the goal of helping people to function better."

Dr. Ellison observes, however, that freedom of inquiry under which scientists have operated is now being challenged by two fears: fear of political abuse and fear that human beings will be altered "in ways that violate human integrity and dignity."

Regarding the first fear, he notes that most present governments are dictatorships and that problems of overpopulation, famine, and economic difficulties may force free nations to become more despotic in the future.

There is no question that sophisticated drugs and electronic treatment can be used by a totalitarian government. Dr. Peter R. Breggin, a Washington psychiatrist and member of the Medical Committee for Human Rights, once told the Senate Health Subcommittee: "If America ever falls to totalitarianism, the dictator will be a behavioral scientist. . . ." Dr. Joseph Caplan, head of psychiatry at Branson Hospital in Toronto, warns that world society may now be on the threshold of a *Brave New World* where people are kept docile with the help of drugs.

"Impossible!" say doubters, who would paraphrase Lincoln: "You can control all the people some of the time; you can even control some of the people all the time; but you can never control all of the people all of the time." Indeed no dictator has ever before controlled all his subjects. *Before* is the catch word. No dictator, not even Hitler, ever had access to the tools for engineering man which exist today.

The second fear, cited by Ellison, harks back to the nature of man as defined by the Bible. Do some brain therapies go too far? Again, most psychiatrists will say that their own wisdom and the controls of society prevent this. But they are speaking of practitioners (even non-Christians) who are influenced by the Judeo-Christian ethic on the value of man, and who work in a society that is free because it is rooted in a biblical faith which champions human rights.

Already, influential voices are saying that crime, violence, threat of war, and other human miseries make it necessary to move beyond individualism. Most heralded is Harvard's B.F. Skinner who believes that scientists can design a world by genetic and behavioral engineering where there will be no wars, overpopulation, starvation, or deprivation.

Few scientists will go so far. Yet a few years ago, Dr. Kenneth B. Clark, then president of the American Psychological Association, called for new drugs to eliminate inhumanity. He suggested that antihostility drugs might be given regularly to national leaders to curb aggressive impulses and prevent them from making war. Fancy world dictators lining up for that! Clark also recommended that the general population might be "psychologically disarmed" by drug therapy, although he denied having in mind the creation of a society of robots.

Evangelical scientists tend to dismiss Skinner's behaviorism as impractical and unattainable. "He doesn't give enough credit to the spontaneous processes in human thinking and activity," says Dr. Donald MacKay, an English brain physiologist who frequently speaks to Christian academics. "He's putting too much faith into experience based on his work with simple animals."

D. Gareth Jones, an anatomist at the University of Western Australia, thinks present neurobiological developments do "not justify reactionary cries of alarm. We are surrounded by individuals suffering from defects of one sort or another; the remedy of these defects and the alleviation of suffering are cardinal principles of medicine which apply as much in modern biological medicine as in more traditional medicine." Jones cautions that "A line must be drawn, however, between this approach and that which attempts to *improve* man according to unspecified goals." The Australian evangelical further fears that the search for the "ideal man" could lead to the "dehumanization of man" (*Journal of the American Scientific Affiliation,* December 1974, p. 153). Along this line, the late Dr. Albert Schweitzer, a religious liberal, once remarked, "The more man becomes superman, the more inhuman he becomes" (Allen R. Utke, *Bio-Babel,* John Knox Press, p. 219).

Variety of Responses

Many evangelicals are not well informed about the latest therapies in mental health and the possible consequences of current research. Their attitudes toward psychiatry range from outright hostility to enthusiastic acceptance of therapies which do not clearly violate Christian principles.

Hostility is most keenly felt by Christian psychiatrists in the U.S. Bible Belt where some pastors naively link current practice with outdated Freudian methods. Only about 10 percent of the 27,000 U.S. psychiatrists are admittedly Freudian.

These pastor-critics preach a Bible-and-prayer therapy for most mental illness and ascribe severe cases to demon possession. They fail to recognize a complexity of causes in mental illness.

Dr. Jay Adams of Westminister Theological Seminary studied the mental health scene and concluded that secular psychology and psychiatry fail to solve mankind's problems because nonbiblical principles are being applied. Adams developed a counseling methodology based wholly on the Bible which he calls "nouthetic counseling." This method is now widely used by evangelical pastors and some professional counselors.

Nouthetic counseling generally follows this procedure: First, the counselor helps his client sort out his problems. Second, they consult the Scripture together to see what God has to say about the problems. Third, the counselor shows the counselee how his difficulties have resulted from his failure to live according to God's plan. Fourth, the counselor proposes practical assignments which he believes will help the person redirect his life according to God's will as expressed in the Bible.

Nouthetic counselors claim this method quickly gets to the basic causes of many problems such as worry, fear, depression, addiction to drugs, interpersonal difficulties at work, marriage conflicts, and parent-child difficulties. They refer patients with obvious organic diseases to physicians.

With the growing popularity of nouthetic counseling, a tension has developed between these counselors and some Christian psychiatrists who say the method is too simplistic. The nouthetic counselors lambast the psychiatrists for not dealing directly with spiritual factors.

Christian psychiatrists readily admit that spiritual forces are involved, along with physical and psychological factors. Under physical factors, Dr. David Busby of Park Ridge, Ill. lists heredity, blows to the head, infections or poisoning of the brain and nervous system, brain tumors, alcohol, narcotics, etc. Psychological forces may include excessive anxiety, guilt, and fears, many of which stem from bad childhood experiences. Spiritual forces, he says, can be direct attacks of Satan and the natural consequences of sin.

Some evangelicals have confidence only in Christian psychiatrists, citing 1 Corinthians 2:14: "A natural man does not accept the things of the Spirit of God: for they are foolishness unto him, and he cannot understand them, because they are spiritually appraised." They fear unbelieving psychiatrists will try to tear down their faith, perhaps even blaming it for their illness. This has happened. Psychiatric patients at Wilson Hospital in Johnson City, N.Y. for example, have reportedly been forbidden to watch "The PTL Club" on television. Dr. Q.D.

Schubmehl claims the program makes patients think they can get better through faith alone.

A growing number of evangelicals recognize that both the causes and cures of mental illness defy simplicity. They see that just as a variety of agents brings an individual to the breaking point, so a variety of persons and therapies must be involved in the healing process. They believe that all healing is from God. Family, fellow Christians, pastors, and professional therapists are God's agents through whom He *usually* chooses to work. But if the patient is to be helped, he must surrender to God's care and commitment and begin following principles of good mental health expressed in the Bible and suggested by Christian professionals.

These knowledgeable evangelicals are also aware that normal, rational human emotions have a proper place in life. Anger, fear, anxiety, disappointment, elation, excitement, and happiness should be felt in appropriate circumstances. Frequently, God speaks to us through negative emotions. There is no virtue in absolute tranquility, they say, nor should it be sought in drugs.

Theologian Vernon Grounds stated, "That a person can be emotionally improved while he remains ethically and spiritually unimproved." Conversely, "from a Christian viewpoint, emotional health is not an end in itself; at best it is a means to the end of living life to the glory of God. . . . Precisely for this reason," wrote Grounds, "evangelicalism insists that no therapy is adequate unless it ultimately helps a man to relate himself to God through faith in Jesus Christ (*His*, October 1963, pp. 25-26).

This better understanding of mental illness and therapies has led to the upgrading of counseling and psychology departments in Christian colleges and seminaries. Pastors are trained in counseling procedures and taught when to refer a counselee to someone with more skills. Correspondingly, numbers of Christian psychiatrists and psychologists have set up group practices in Atlanta, Chattanooga, Chicago, and other cities. A few local congregations even sponsor professional counseling centers where a patient may receive needed therapy for a fee dependent on his income.

These combined efforts have resulted in a broader understanding of delinquency and criminality. A Yale University study, for example, of

78 "violent" teen delinquents in a reform school disclosed that 96 percent had neurological abnormalities (memory lapses, histories of blackouts, dizzy spells, dreamlike states, anxiety attacks, and hallucinations), and that three of four had been seriously abused by parents or guardians.

Mental illness in the U.S. has become an epidemic. About 40 percent of *all* hospital beds in the U.S. are occupied by persons with mental problems. A half million persons enter mental hospitals every year. An astounding 37 million Americans spend $2.5 billion annually on psychoactive drug prescriptions to relieve anxiety, tension, insomnia, etc. Two billion dollars more is spent on illegal drugs which also affect the brain and nervous system.

Christians must become informed and face issues relating to research in brain physiology and developments in mental health care. We must also show intelligent concern for the mentally ill.

8

Christian Perspectives on Brain Research and Treatment of the Mentally Ill

DR. ROGER VEITH, NEUROSURGEON

The neurosurgeon is held in more awe than most doctors because his everyday work is with the brain. Dr. Veith is himself in awe of the mysteries of the brain, an awe which led him to first begin thinking seriously about God.

"I grew up in a little northern Illinois town. Although I thought it was nice to go to church, religion never made any impact on my life. I wanted to do right morally, but didn't really believe there was a God who loved me and would direct my path. It was not until my first year in medical school that I decided there had to be a Designer, an Organizer.

"I was dissecting cadavers ten hours a day, and was overwhelmed with the complexity of the human body and the biochemistry, physiology, and neuroanatomy of the brain with its 15 billion cells working in such perfect harmony. It seemed easier to believe that one could throw up millions of letters and have them come down in the order of the

Encyclopedia Britannica than to think the brain had developed by accident.

"As I worked on the cadaver, I also thought, *This guy was alive and now he's dead. What happened to him? What will happen to me when I die?*

"Seeking an understanding of God and the Bible, I ran into the Inter-Varsity Christian Fellowship at Duke. For a while I thought they were out of their minds—fanatics, freaks. But after struggling for several months, I got down on my knees and said, 'Lord, I don't know who You are, but I know You exist. I don't know the Bible, and I don't understand it all. I just know there *is* a God, and You must be the One. Come into my life.' Nothing dramatic happened, though I certainly felt I had found the purpose I was here for. Very gradually, God worked with me. A minister discipled me for five or six years. He met with me every Saturday morning. I came to trust in Christ as my Saviour and to more deeply understand God's claims on my life."

Dr. Veith found "everything tremendously exciting" in medical school. "I couldn't get enough of it." The last two years he felt drawn to some type of surgery. He thought this might be general surgery, then thoracic surgery. During his internship he settled on neurosurgery.

"The brain fascinated me. After 13 years of practice it still does, especially all the unknowns. For instance, we can precisely locate the controls for many physical functions. We know, for example, that the control for the right thumb is in the most posterior part of the frontal lobe of the brain called the precentral gyrus. We can stimulate the medial temporal lobe, which is a big area, and the patient recollects sensations, emotions, feelings he's had before. *Deja vu,* the feeling you have when you walk into a strange room and sense you have been there before, originates in this area. We know a lot about the anatomy and the structures of the brain. But composites of brain activity—memory, thought processes, calculations, assumptions, judgments, decisions—well, we're not really very sure how these things happen.

"From a scientific standpoint we just know very little about the intangibles that make man a unique, spiritual being. We know that consciousness depends on the reticular activating system which is in the upper part of the brain stem. Essentially, it keeps firing messages to the cortex which is where you do your thinking and decision-making. But we can't locate the soul, the image of God. In my judgment, it would have to be somewhere in that rational part of the being that allows you to make a choice.''

Dr. Veith is humble in speaking about how the image of God is expressed in man. "How can I say it adequately? There are so many facets. It's the capacity you have to look up to God, to worship, to seek wisdom from God. The capacity for honesty, kindness, empathy in reaching out to other people. The capacity to look at another individual, not just in a cold, scientific, medical way, but also in a loving, caring way, to accept him not just for what he is, but for what he might become as well.

"When I have a patient, I unconditionally accept that patient and try to do what I can, the best I can. I can't cut corners on him. There are a lot of things I can do medically and a lot of things I can't do, but I can always have a part in a patient's life, and his family's, when I allow the image of God in me to reflect to all those around me.''

Dr. Veith believes there are cases which may call for psychosurgery: "obsessive, compulsive personalities that are just basket cases, people with terrible pain from terminal cancer or crush injuries, for example. Psychosurgery can be a very effective operation when done the right way. With radio frequency and thermal coagulation, the surgeon can dissect a very small portion of the brain and alleviate a lot of difficulties.

"No question," he says, "but that you can destroy part of the brain and practically change the personality. To think of psychosurgery as something done routinely, done to control other people, is fiction.

"Drugs, which are not my field, probably hold greater possibilities for changing personalities. They can be administered on a much wider scale than surgery.

"In the 18th century the Germans found they could cure some illnesses with drugs. They thought they'd find a drug pretty soon that would cure *all* illnesses. Time has not borne out their optimism. I suspect we're in the same sort of situation now with biochemical drugs for the brain, looking for the ultimate answer.''

To build or transplant a brain seems to Dr. Veith "physically impossible. You'd have to put it all together in about three-and-a-half minutes and give it a blood supply.

"We've concluded that most brain cells, when they are destroyed or are deprived of their oxidized blood supply, do not regenerate. There is laboratory evidence that possibly some do. Even so, regeneration doesn't happen at a high enough level to be clinically significant."

He thinks man's sinful nature and ego-tripping may play a role in some of the search for panaceas, for immortality. "Don't get me wrong, I'm not against progress, but I have to be aware that many 'solutions' have turned out to be harmful—all the carcinogens we are getting from chemicals, for example. Still, in science and medicine, we go on playing the money game, the power game, the position game."

His philosophy about risky brain surgery flows from a spiritual commitment made in medical school. "I have to believe that God has a role in everything I do. Jesus said, 'Without Me you can do nothing.' That is very real to me. So I say, 'God, You have a role in this, so I want You to guide me. I'm weak without You.' No matter how strong I might be, how confident, I know there are so many things I can't control; so I can't make any kind of guarantee. There's an awful lot that I have to leave to the Lord."

DR. TRUMAN ESAU, PSYCHIATRIST

Dr. Esau practices psychiatry in a sophisticated Chicago suburb. He is concerned that Christians who once were distrustful of psychology and psychiatry may now be leaning too far in the other direction.

"I'm troubled about the pop psychiatry as presented in some Christian books. I see this as a superficial attempt to say that psychology and the Bible really aren't very far apart. There is no more a Christian psychology than a Christian auto repair. The only way there could be a Christian psychology is if all emotional problems had a spiritual origin. And I don't think that can be said, because it leads to oversimplification of the problems which people have."

Dr. Esau himself holds to a "traditional Christian view" about the nature of man. "Man is much more than a body, I believe. He is at base a spiritual being with a spiritual nature and conscience. The human experience requires the body and the mind for expression. If there is an impairment in the brain, there is an impairment in human relationships and perceptions of life.

"I see consciousness as a function of the brain. What's the relationship between consciousness and the soul? Where does the soul reside? I don't know. As a scientist I can't answer, and biblically I can't answer either, except that man is a living soul."

Spiritual health doesn't guarantee mental health and vice versa, Dr. Esau says. "One can be schizophrenic and still have a right attitude toward God. I don't deny that the schizophrenia will alter the experience with God. But it may not alter the genuineness of the relationship.

"I am certainly not a behaviorist as B.F. Skinner and some others claim to be. They think of man as superconditioned to respond to certain stimuli. Behaviorism is a much more narrow definition.

"Skinner doesn't talk about sin. Of course, there is no sin if man is only a conditioned animal. It's only when you see man as having a spiritual nature and a conscience that you can talk about sin. What is sin? Violation of relationship with God. Sinning against one's brother or against one's self is also sinning against God. We can participate in sin without being conscious of it. When one is aware that he is violating a relationship, sin has greater significance.

"There's no such thing as a 'violence gene,'" Dr. Esau declares. "The legal pleading of insanity is greatly overdone in criminal law today. It is very important that a person come to accept his own level of responsibility for his difficulties, whether he's charged with a crime or not. He can only change as he accepts responsibility. That is a crucial concept, and much more therapeutic as time goes along, particularly in the context of family therapy.

"In some ways the development of psychology as a profession has resulted from the church defaulting in its responsibility of caring for people. The church has become less and less the place where relationships are nurtured. It has become more and more superficial, and often does not deal with people where they really are.

"The evangelical church is especially weak in ministry to families. It sometimes even adds to the fragmentation of the family by having separate programs for family members. Family togetherness cannot be accomplished just by sitting together in morning worship. No preacher is able to meet all of their needs simultaneously.

"I would like to see the church build more programs for the family. Let families participate together, and experience each other. Show the dirty laundry to some extent, and then help each other. People yearn for this all the time. Some churches divide into home fellowships. That was the way in the primitive church—people worshiped as families.

"Supporting, caring relationships in the family and in the church contribute immeasurably to emotional health. What is a healthy person? One who is aware of his own feelings, one who knows what is going on in relationships, one whose system of defenses supports his being honest and open, rather than supporting deceit and self-concealment. Unfortunately, much of conservative Christianity supports people in covering up rather than in being open.

"You hear, 'Pray about it and it will go away.' That's a misunderstanding of the Bible. If you pray about it, you will become more aware of what the problem is, so that you can deal with it. Otherwise you're just putting it under the rug."

Dr. Esau is distressed by the escalating use of prescription drugs. "I think it's criminal the way tranquilizers are prescribed. These drugs have become the middle-class substitute for alcohol.

"Mark it down partly to drug company salesmanship and partly to a cop-out on the part of the doctor. He gives a drug, the patient feels better, and so the doctor assumes he has helped him. But what if the patient becomes addicted to that drug?

"I believe in medications for acute situations to help a person get in touch with reality. Sure, I'll give them, but not permanently."

Dr. Esau thinks there are "circumstances in which shock treatment can be life-saving. But it's very rare—I haven't used shock treatment in two or three years—and I think it's overdone. Sometimes, though, if the alternative is suicide, you have to do it.

"Psychosurgery for psychiatric disorders is of little use in clinical psychiatry. Besides, you have to look at the value question when you dig inside the human brain. I've never recommended surgery for mental illness.

"Mental illness is a big problem in this country. The present federal community health program is nearly bankrupt, as far as helping people in depth. A little bit for everybody is what it amounts to.

"Government bureaucracy can't cure all mental illness. Some state psychiatric hospitals are as bad as prisons. I wouldn't want to be part of that system, because I don't see any way to change it. Still, you can't assume that the present private establishments are sufficient for dealing with the problems either.

"I'm encouraged by churches involved with ministries that get people in touch with themselves and others. Some evangelical congregations are doing an excellent job in this area. LaSalle Street Church in Chicago, for example, is a small congregation; yet they have a professionally staffed counseling center.

"Not every church can do this. But churches can at least be aware of needs and start to do something."

9

Homosexuality: Sin, Sickness, or Choice?

The election is over in Miami. The gays have lost and are angry. Their target was Anita Bryant, the Florida orange juice lady and devout Christian, who led the successful campaign to keep known homosexuals from teaching in Dade County schools. Now she is speaking in Scope Arena in Norfolk, Virginia to citizens concerned about homosexuals.

A noisy crowd is outside. Militant gays wave banners before TV cameras: "Say No to Bigotry," "Stop Anita Bryant," "Defend Lesbian Mothers." Police keep them away from about 150 church people who proclaim: "Gays Are Godless" and "Sinners, not sickness."

Polarization

The demonstrations indicate the sharpness of the controversy in America today, where gays claim 10 percent of the population.

The fight goes on. "Today it is the gay community, tomorrow it may be the left-handed people," cries Rims Barber, an official of the American Civil Liberties Union (Quoted UPI, June 9, 1977). "Homosexuality is not a civil rights problem,'' counters singer Pat Boone in an open letter to Los Angeles Mayor Tom Bradley. "Being black, Chinese, or Jewish is an act of God. Being homosexual is an abomination to God.'' (*Christian Life,* November 1977, p. 25).

The bitter divisions and polarizing opinions run through every segment of Western society. Psychiatrists haggle over definitions of homosexuality. The American Psychiatric Association declared officially in 1973 that "By itself homosexuality does not necessarily constitute a psychiatric disorder.'' The vote to adopt was by no means unanimous, and many in the profession strongly disagree.

In 1977 the annual meeting of the American Bar Association featured an acrimonious panel debate between gays and straights. John V. Briggs, a California legislator, termed homosexuals "unstable,'' "anti-life,'' "moral dropouts'' and "a self-styled minority like wife-beaters and ex-convicts.'' Briggs wants a law in his state that will allow any school board to fire teachers "who engage in public homosexual conduct.'' E. Carrington Boggan, a New York attorney and admitted homosexual, shot back that homosexuals were as "stable'' as heterosexuals and said he could cite a number of gay couples who have lived together for 20 and 30 years. Boggan argued that the same rationale that would reject homosexuals as teachers would exclude persons who held different religious and political beliefs from their parents.

Church Opinions

Major Protestant denominations have been wrangling for a decade over moral definitions of homosexuality and whether or not gays should be ordained into the ministry. Official reports and decisions vary and are often contradictory. For example, delegates to the 1978 assembly of the Presbyterian Church in America (Southern) refused to classify homosexuality as sin and by majority vote declared only that the condition "falls short of God's plan'' for sexual practice. In 1977 the American Lutheran Church accepted a committee's decision that homosexuality is sin, but said gays should not be denied civil rights and should be accepted into church membership. Episcopalian authorities, after prolonged debate at their 1979 General Convention forbade the ordination of homosexuals as priests.

Divergent views are frequently held by leaders within the same denomination. Episcopalian Bishop Paul Moore of New York ordained an avowed lesbian, while Bishop Bennett J. Sims of the Georgia diocese said he would not. Bishop Sims calls "the steady drift toward a sanction of homosexuality an ill wind blowing through society and the church." The question, he says, is "how to regard homosexuality as an amenable personality disorder, which is how I view it, and yet insist upon a true and loving regard for persons" (Address to Episcopal Diocese of Atlanta, 1978).

The issue is further confused by the emergence of gay churches in almost every large American city. Some claim to follow evangelical doctrine; others are more liberally oriented. Gay forms of worship are much like those of straights. They have Sunday Schools and baptisms, sing hymns, take offerings, and listen to sermons. A visitor will notice two differences between straight and gay churches. There are few children at gay services, and after church, men go home with men and women with women.

Until about five years ago, conservative evangelicals generally ignored the gay challenge. Pastors preached against homosexuality only in the context of other sins which God condemns. Sunday School teachers rarely mentioned it. Families didn't talk about it. The subject was low on the agenda of evangelical pastors' conferences.

A series of bizarre sex crimes combined with a gay drive for public recognition and full rights for practicing homosexuals awakened evangelicals. Suddenly, homosexual roles blossomed in television dramas with gays portrayed as normal or as persecuted by straights.

The militant gays became darlings of the liberal media and entertainment world, which saw them as an oppressed minority being held down by self-righteous, Bible-thumping straights. Thousands of closet homosexuals went public, proclaiming themselves proud to be gays. Never in modern times had gays been so bold and flagrant in their conduct.

Then came the battle of Miami with Anita Bryant risking her career and even her life to keep public and private schools from being forced to hire practicing homosexuals as teachers.

Evangelical publishers broke the wall of silence. The first books on the subject didn't sell well. The first articles in Christian magazines brought some nasty letters, along with others saying it was time Christians began speaking out. Some of the autobiographical stories shocked readers who hadn't imagined that professing Christians could be involved in such gross sin: Young adults, products of evangelical churches and schools, told about their battles with homosexuality.

A Presbyterian minister, raised in Youth for Christ, president of his high school Bible club, graduate of an evangelical college and seminary, and married to a Christian girl, described how he became involved with homosexuals. A lesbian recalled how she had been raised in a "strict" Christian home. Most stories had happy endings, with the homosexuals finding deliverance through Jesus Christ. Some defended the gay lifestyle, as two anonymous gays, both alumni of noted evangelical schools, were allowed to, in *Christian Life* magazine:

> The fact is, some Christians happen to be homosexual. It is time that all Christians, straight and gay, affirm the sanctity of intimate, committed personal relationships. The Bible is not a collection of proof-texts to prove or disprove our cultural presuppositions and subcultural prejudices. It is time that all Christians, straight and gay, begin to take seriously the careful study of God's Word (*Christian Life*, October 1978, p. 57).

Where Do We Draw the Line?

As the so-called gay revolution continues, many evangelicals are confused, and divided on questions regarding gay rights.

● Where is the line to be drawn for gays in employment and housing, if at all?
● How far should a Christian worker go in trying to help gays?
● Should a church receive known homosexuals into membership?
● And most difficult of all, how shall we confront the gay influence and challenge to society? Is it sickness, sin, or choice?

Homosexuality and the Bible

We cannot intelligently deal with these questions until we understand the condition of homosexuality. Homosexuality was never God's intention in Creation. He created our first parents Adam and Eve, male and female, a beautiful diversity, not Adam and George or Eve and Doris

(Gen. 1:27). He established heterosexual marriage: "Therefore shall a man leave his father and his mother, and shall cleave unto his wife: and they shall be one flesh"—a beautiful unity of contrasting sexual beings (Gen. 2:24, KJV). Sexual relationships that violate this principle "miss the mark" (the meaning of *sin* in Romans 3:23) and "fall short of the glory of God."

There was undoubtedly homosexuality long before Sodom, but this is the first time it is evident in the biblical record. Sodom was probably not much different from Castro Street and the Haight-Ashbury section in modern San Francisco or Greenwich Village in New York City. Homosexual hustlers roamed the streets looking for new conquests. Upon hearing that two good-looking strangers were visiting Lot, they surrounded the house and demanded that Lot "bring them out unto us, that we may know them" (Gen. 19:5, KJV). The rest of the story in Genesis 19 is well known to Bible students.

Some gay interpreters try to twist this episode in unbelievable fashion, saying that the sins of the Sodomites were inhospitality and rape, not homosexuality. "That we may know them," they say, indicates only a desire for social companionships. Then why did Lot call their intentions wicked? Why were they willing to break down the door to be hospitable to strangers? Why did Lot feel constrained to offer his daughters, if he did not believe his guests were in danger of homosexual rape? Leaving these questions aside, it should be enough to note that "know" was a common Hebrew euphemism for sexual intercourse.

These gays admit that the Mosaic Law condemned homosexuality. (See Leviticus 18:22, 24, 30; 20:13.) They claim such condemnation does not apply to homosexual relationships today for two reasons: (1) God opposed homosexuality so as to promote population growth in Israel; (2) The Law is fulfilled in Christ. They also argue that if the prohibition against homosexuality stands today, then Christians should observe the dietary rules of the Law along with regulations relating to sex, and should stone adulterers and homosexuals.

The first reason cited is obviously ridiculous. The second is at best a half-truth. Christ did fulfill the Law, but moral standards remain. Adultery, for example, was wrong before the Law was given. So was homosexuality. Stoning for sexual misconduct could apply only in a theocracy such as Israel. We live in a secular state, although many of our laws are rooted in Judeo-Christian morality.

Some gays claim that the friendship of David and Jonathan proves that God sanctioned homosexual relationships. Their conclusions are defamatory and border on the absurd. There is no hint of a sexual relationship in the biblical account. The obscure Hebrew word in 1 Samuel 20:41 (KJV) translated "exceeded" in King James does not mean *orgasm*, but "wept still more" than Jonathan over their parting.

One would think that gays who claim to accept the Bible as authoritative would bow before Romans 1:26-27: "For this cause God gave them over to degrading passions; for their women exchanged the natural function for that which is unnatural, and in the same way also the men abandoned the natural function of the woman and burned in their desire toward one another, men with men committing indecent acts and receiving in their own persons the due penalty for their error."

Some gays call this passage cultural baggage of the first century. Paul, they say, was merely using an illustration from the pagan world to prove that all have sinned. They say this passage belongs with those forbidding women to cut their hair and speak in the assembly. Other gays take a different tack! The sinners of Romans 1, were really heterosexuals who were violating their sexual norms by participating in homosexual acts.

There were certainly homosexuals in the New Testament congregations along with other sinners, whom Paul considered unworthy of the kingdom of God. (See 1 Corinthians 6:9-10.) "Such were some of you," he reminded the Corinthian believers, "but you were washed, but you were sanctified, but you were justified in the name of the Lord Jesus, and in the Spirit of our God" (6:11). Were these believers ever tempted to return to their old lifestyles? Yes. They could take comfort in the promise: "No temptation has overtaken you but such as is common to man; and God is faithful, who will not allow you to be tempted beyond what you are able; but with the temptation will provide the way of escape also, that you may be able to endure it" (1 Cor. 10:13).

The modern apologists will not give up. Defenders of homosexual practice and premarital and extramarital sex speak loftily of love being the highest authority. In July 1977, a United Church of Christ committee claimed that concern for another determines moral rightness. This is the old song of situation ethics, the self-exaltation of modern existentialism. The "I" decides what is loving and what is not. No absolutes here. No scriptural authority recognizing that truth and love are not in opposition.

The gay churches are well organized. The Metropolitan Community Church alone has about 80 gay congregations in major U.S. cities, and is larger than some small evangelical denominations. The gay churches are assisted by at least 10 parachurch groups who teach that homosexuals can have valid sexual relationships. A gay caucus is active in most mainline American denominations.

Gays have conferences and camps just like straight evangelicals. Ten homosexually oriented groups sponsored a conference at Kirkbridge, a popular Christian retreat center near Bangor, Pennsylvania. One of the main speakers was Malcolm Boyd, author of several best-selling religious books before "coming out." Boyd, an Episcopal priest, likened his emergence from the closet with "being born again."

The principal speaker, Jesuit priest John J. McNeill, told the conferees:

God so created human nature that a certain percentage of men and women always and everywhere develop as homosexuals. Thus the homosexual condition is according to God's created plan. It has no necessary connection with sin, failure, or sickness. It is another way of being human. Homosexuals bring particular gifts, qualities, and talents . . . to human society. . . . The love that exists between homosexuals, granted that it is a constructive human love . . . is not sinful nor does it alienate the lovers from God" (Quoted by AP, May 3, 1977).

Physical Bases for Homosexuality

Some people believe that homosexuality is biologically and/or culturally determined and thus represents a God-given sexual orientation. This is widely disputed by psychiatric authorities, who say that homosexuality results from a myriad of factors and that few cases are the same.

A small number of persons are born sexually abnormal because of genetic defects. One example is testicular feminization: The XY chromosomes clearly say male, but no sex organs are in view. The testes are recessed where the uterus might be in a normal female. In the past most of these babies passed as girls. Some decided that they were lesbians and never married. Some did marry and tried to get pregnant. Unable to do so, they consulted a doctor who discovered the problem. Because such a condition indicates a greatly increased chance of cancer, doctors often recommend that the incomplete sex organs be surgically removed.

A second genetic oddity results in a chromosomal female with male sex organs. A third produces a hermaphrodite with some combination of male and female organs. A fourth defect results in a male that looks like a female because of an inherited insensitivity to masculinizing hormones. According to Professor John Money at John Hopkins Medical Center, such persons may function as sexually normal females, even though every cell in their body carries the male XY chromosomal complement.

Scientists know that the hypothalamus, a tiny organ at the base of the brain, is the agent in sex development. It releases a hormone that stimulates the pituitary gland to secrete other hormones which, in turn, spur the sex glands to produce gonads (testes in normal males and ovaries in females). The gonads secrete the critical sex hormones: androgens in males and estrogens and progesterones in females. These sex hormones cause the respective male and female organs to develop, and further stimulate secondary sexual characteristics.

This much is generally known. But research into the biological processes that result in sexual differentiation is inconclusive at many points.

Social and Emotional Bases

The great majority of homosexuals cannot justify their lifestyle with the plea, "I was born this way." Their claim that a genetic defect indicates that homosexual practice is God's plan for a person makes no sense. We might as well say that God made a young man a hemophiliac so that he might practice bleeding.

This is not to say victims of genetically caused sexual disorders do not deserve compassion. They do, along with sufferers from other inherited diseases. Sex-change operations which can help them lead more normal lives should not be denied any more than we would withhold treatment for persons with hemophilia or cystic fibrosis.

Biology, however, is not the major defense of most practicing homosexuals for their lifestyle. They plead cultural determination, a catch-all term that includes a disparity of unfortunate happenings in childhood.

A gay businessman in Tennessee, father of two children, recalls that he was raped as a boy by a bachelor neighbor. A lesbian from another state painfully remembers her mother saying, "I was so certain you'd be a boy, I don't even have a name for you." Robert became Roberta. The girl's father was abusive and her steady tried to rape her at 16. She came to despise sex.

Every counselor hears such stories. Dr. Toby Rieber, a psychiatrist and coauthor of a book on male homosexuality, has never found a good father-son relationship in studying backgrounds of male gays.

Still, childhood traumas do not provide sufficient reason for a lifestyle that is condemned in the Bible. For every gay who laments, "I can't help the way I am," there are two straights who suffered parental abuse and traumatic sexual mishaps and are now living normal, heterosexual lives.

Those who feel preconditioned to homosexuality are the most vulnerable to gay hustlers. A Tennessee businessman lived a normal married life until about age 40. He taught Sunday School and was a good father to his children. He felt homosexual inclinations, but fought them off until being "picked up" by a gay business associate. Unwilling to give up his lover, he wrecked his business and his marriage and is today part of the gay world.

The girl whose mother had wanted a boy needed a mother. She suppressed her "crush" on a woman teacher, dated men, and experienced two tragic marriages to men she didn't love. After her second divorce, she chose to live with gay women, but this life did not meet her deepest needs. She drank heavily (homosexuals are three times more likely than straights to be heavy drinkers) and often flew into insane rages. Finally she decided to end her tortured life. On her way to the kitchen to turn on the gas jets, she fell on her knees and cried, "God forgive me! God, forgive me!" She had heard the Gospel as a child and a few weeks before had been witnessed to by a friend. In her despair she accepted Christ as her Saviour.

Loneliness soon drove her back to the gay life. It was the suicide of a dear friend that impelled her to make Christ the Lord of her life. This time she broke forever with what she knew was sin. She is today striving to win gays to repent of their sin and trust in Christ.

Spokesmen for militant gay organizations claim that gays cannot change. The facts do not support this. Sex researchers Masters and Johnson, who can by no means be called antigay, report a 65 percent "conversion" rate among 67 gay men and women patients who wanted to live heterosexually. Psychiatrists' statistics, reports Dr. James D. Mallory, reveal that 30 to 66 percent of all homosexuals who come for treatment, whether with a Christian psychiatrist or not, are cured. The key to change, as with alcoholism, is motivation and faith.

Gay Power

Today's militant homosexuals try to suppress these figures. They want to be seen as an oppressed minority, no more able to change their status than blacks or Hispanics. They crusade for public endorsement of their lifestyle. They march in parades, lobby in Congress and state legislatures, demonstrate at church conferences, foster gay clubs on campuses, and pressure mayors and governors to set aside a time as "Gay Pride Week."

To homosexuals with doubts and misgivings about the gay life, they declare: "You cannot change. Learn to accept the way you are."

There are large gay communities in every major city (up to a quarter of the population in San Francisco, which is now recruiting homosexual policemen), and many admitted gays are in state legislatures. Two assistants to Boston's Mayor Kevin White are proudly gay. Gays take credit for electing a number of mayors, including the mayor of Washington, D.C. They have clout in Congress. Forty Congressmen have formed a coalition to promote gay rights.

The American media is sensitive to gay power. Major book publishers, newspapers, and magazines tread softly. Unofficial gay censors, inside and outside of media organizations, abound.

Gays are trying to get veto power over radio and television station licenses. They intend to see that no station can renew its government license without approval from their representatives. Stations are pressured to drop evangelists who dare preach that homosexuality is sin. Their most notable success has come in Dallas where evangelist James Robison's contract was cancelled by WFAA-TV on gay allegations that he had violated the FCC's "Fairness Doctrine."

Gays are strongest in the entertainment industry where they can virtually ruin the career of any actor or entertainer who dares oppose them. Ask Anita Bryant, whom homosexuals acknowledge as Enemy Number One. She directs a counseling service for gays and has repeatedly said she does not hate homosexuals but only wishes to keep them from infringing on the rights of parents who do not want their children taught by gays. Yet,

- Singer Rod McKuen announced, "If she continues (opposing gay rights), I intend to call upon every comedian friend I know to have so many jokes go forth about her throughout the land that she will be a laughingstock such as this country has never seen before." (Quoted by AP, May 3, 1977.) (He hasn't succeeded: In 1978 Anita was voted "Most Admired Woman" by readers of *Good Housekeeping* magazine, ahead of Rosalyn Carter, Betty Ford, Lady Bird Johnson, and Queen Elizabeth. *The Ladies Home Journal* poll for "Women of the Year" in effect blackballed Anita by selecting the women for which readers could vote.)
- When she was to appear in New Orleans, the chairman of the local AFTRA (American Federation of Radio and Television Artists) asked local radio-TV members to deny her their assistance. This was unprecedented in the history of the union.
- Anita and husband Bob Green constantly receive bomb and death threats. All their mail is x-rayed.

In contending that professed homosexuals should not be allowed to teach in schools, Anita is backed by many mental health professionals. Children in junior high school, they note, are already confused enough in trying to establish sexual identity. Homosexual teachers will only compound this difficulty.

Advertised homosexuals are already teaching in many school systems. The San Francisco School Board voted 7-0 to approve inclusion of gay lifestyles studies in high school sex education classes. The San Francisco Gay Teachers Alliance now want gay studies taught at elementary grade levels. Also in San Francisco, in spite of union protests, public mental health workers, even clerks and typists, have been forced to watch homosexual activities in films to "sensitize" them for dealing with gay clients.

Approval of homosexuality as a lifestyle has been creeping into high school sociology and psychology textbooks. Two such books were rejected by the Texas State Board of Education, and another was withdrawn by the publisher, after textbook analyst Norma Gabler objected. She quoted this paragraph from the text, *Our Psychological World* (Prentice-Hall, p. 37):

This process is called "sex-role development" and means that we are trained gradually in the ways of behavior as a male or female. Put another way, we learn how to be a man or a woman sexually and adopt that role—as if we were in a play—until that role becomes second nature.

Gays are further propagandizing their lifestyle by publishing biographical studies of famous homosexuals in history. One book by A.L. Rowse entitled *Homosexuals in History*, (The Macmillan Publishing Co.) claims that such famous figures as Erasmus, Leonardo da Vinci, Michelangelo, Francis Bacon, Frederick the Great, Somerset Maugham, Walt Whitman, Herman Melville, and Nathaniel Hawthorne were homosexuals. A close reading reveals many of the judgments were made from scanty circumstantial evidence. Some gays even claim that Jesus was a homosexual.

Reactions to Gay Power

However, gay power is not as great as it might seem. The movement has suffered a number of referendum defeats on the teacher issue since Miami. The Pennsylvania legislature rebuked their state's governor for proclaiming a "Gay Pride Week." Millions of Americans are joining Anita Bryant, Jerry Falwell, James Robison and others in crusades for morality.

This is in part a backlash to news of gay exploitation, perversion, and in some cases murder of children.

- Almost 100 boys were lured to their death by gay perverts in Texas, California, and Illinois.
- Los Angeles officials report over 30,000 young boys are abused every year by homosexuals, including $1,000-a-day boy prostitutes.
- Gays in Coral Gables, Florida bought into a private school and, through connections with homosexual social workers, offered boarding school scholarships to delinquent and dependent boys, who were then used by homosexuals.
- In Tennessee an Episcopal priest was charged with operating a boys' school for homosexual and pornographic purposes.
- In Traverse City, Michigan homosexuals reportedly organized a church and other "charities" to get tax money and tax-exempt donations for a camp where young boys were recruited into homosexuality.
- The Minneapolis Civil Rights Board ordered the local Big Brothers organization to hire a homosexual applicant to be a Big Brother; to recruit more gays to be Big Brothers; and not to tell mothers whether a Big Brother assigned to their son was homosexual.

"Respectable" homosexuals decry exploitation of children; yet many of them want gays in positions where they can influence youth. Some gay organizations are also working to lower the legal age of consent for sexual relations to 14.

In the April 27, 1979 *National Review*, William F. Buckley, Jr. quoted from the publication *Gala*, citing the goals of the extremist homosexuals: "It is essential that the gay liberation movement as a whole recognize and fight for the rights of children to control their own bodies, free from the antisexual restraints now imposed upon them by adults and by the institutions adults control—religion, the state, the legal profession, the schools, and the family.

"The ultimate goal of the gay liberation movement . . . is freedom of sexual expression for young people and children. . . . We gain nothing by limiting our defense of homosexual love to consensual sex between adults. It is absurd to charge gay men who share their sexuality with boys as 'child molesters.' . . . Those of us who are struggling for gay rights are, moreover, hypocritical if we limit our demands to the protection of consenting adults.''

Gala expressed its opposition to morals based on the "primitive revelations of the Bible.''

Christian Response

In view of all this, what should be the Christian response? Concerned Christian leaders present these suggestions:

1. Become educated about homosexuality. Recognize that homosexuality in most instances may be caused by a variety of factors and that there are no simple answers. At the same time, be aware that the practice of homosexuality is always a choice.

2. Accept what the Bible says about homosexuality as authoritative. The practice is wrong.

3. Be sensitive to the deep needs of persons caught in the web of homosexuality. Offer friendship without compromise. Witness to Christ's delivering power with compassion. Never violate a confidence.

4. Accept nonpracticing homosexuals into your church just as you would other repentant sinners.

5. Support special ministries to homosexuals, staffed by ex-gays who preach deliverance.

6. Get active politically in opposing the intrusion of homosexual teachers, counselors, and gay propaganda into education and public life. Write letters to key officials stating your stand on issues relating to homosexuality. Work for the election of politicians who stand for biblical morality.

Pastor Tim LaHaye, author of *The Unhappy Gays* thinks that "maybe—just maybe—the possibility of having homosexual role models as school teachers is the alarm buzzer that has awakened sleeping Christians.'' (*Christian Life*, November 1978, p. 64).

7. Above all, understand the difference between the Christian position on homosexuality (and other sins such as adultery) and the world's stance. Dr. Kenneth Gangel, president of Miami Christian College in Florida, puts it well: "The Christian believes in absolute standards of truth, ethics, and morality. To be sure, his interpretation of that absolute

biblical standard at any time and place may be based on faulty exegesis and interpretation. Nevertheless, there are some things in which conservative Christianity has always stood firm.

"The world on the other hand, operates its entire system on the basis of relative truth, relative ethics, and relative morality" (*Christian Life*, January 1978, p. 47).

10

Christian Perspectives on Homosexuality: Sin, Sickness, or Choice?

DR. TRUMAN ESAU, PSYCHIATRIST

"I don't believe homosexuality is biological, but that it is learned within the triad of father-mother-child relationships in the family.

"I disagree with the American Psychiatric stand on it. Homosexuality *is* a mental illness and can be resolved in some instances. There is ample clinical evidence of homosexuals who have converted to heterosexuality. The problem is that few homosexuals want to change because it's tough work, but they can do it.

"I'm concerned about the militancy of homosexuals as a special-interest group. They do have civil rights. But they do not have the right to teach any child their way of life. That's stepping on parents' rights and children's rights."

V. ELVING ANDERSON, GENETICIST

"Homosexuality is complex. There are surely psychological and sociological factors involved. Genetically, the problem has not been studied very thoroughly. The few studies that have been done suggest genetic causes in some cases.

"That there is obviously a learned component makes it difficult to study. You can't tell who has the potential without exposure. You would not want to expose people to a test which would tell whether they have homosexual potential.

"I will accept the possibility that by the nature of their biology some people may be more prone to homosexuality and may find it easier to resort to this relationship. This doesn't mean that they must. Homosexual behavior is not inevitable."

LYNN R. BUZZARD, EXECUTIVE DIRECTOR, CHRISTIAN LEGAL SOCIETY

Lynn Buzzard speaks from a background of studies in theology, morality, and law.

"There are two very easy ways to look at homosexuality. One is to say that it's okay because man is okay and God accepts people where they are. The important thing, according to this view, is not whether something is right or wrong by some moral code, but whether individuals are fulfilling themselves as persons, whether there is a commitment of love in a relationship.

"The other view is that gays are the most despicable creatures on earth and should be run out of town on a rail.

"It seems to me that the Christian cannot accept either of these extreme positions, but must look at homosexuality with both trust and love.

"This requires that we try to understand homosexuality. We find that its causes are not easy to define or separate. Most authorities will say that it is the result of a combination of family influences and personal choice.

"Truth and love also demand that we reexamine our prejudices about homosexuals. The percentage of gays trying to seduce young boys is no greater than the proportion of heterosexuals trying to seduce the opposite sex. The idea that all male homosexuals are effeminate is not true. Some are. Most are not.

The belief that homosexuals are all mental cases is false, although psychiatric studies indicate that gays do have a high level of neuroses and psychoses. We also need to differentiate between the condition and practice of homosexuality. Many who are inclined to homosexual behavior reject such impulses.

"If we hold to the Bible, we'll accept its words as authoritative about homosexual practice. It's incredible the way some gays misinterpret Scripture to justify their lifestyle. One writer who is sympathetic to gays advises them to 'quit trying to twist the Bible—it clearly says homosexuality is wrong.' He's right. The Bible calls homosexuality sin. One Old Testament passage, Deuteronomy 22:5, even says it is an abomination for men to dress as women and women as men.

"Homosexuals are mentioned in the New Testament, along with idolaters, adulterers, drunkards, etc., as being among those who will not inherit the kingdom of God (1 Cor. 6:9-10). In Romans 1 Paul speaks about the wrath of God which falls upon sinners who reject clear knowledge of God's power and deity, refuse to honor Him, and follow unnatural functions. (See Romans 1:21-32.)

"Some say homosexuality is a cultural thing, like forbidding women to cut their hair or to speak in the church. This is hard to believe. The biblical writers present homosexuality as wrong, along with other practices that are clearly sins, not social or cultural customs. The case is even stronger when you consider the theology of marriage and family. God created man and woman as complements for each other. Union with the same sex makes no sense in the context of the mutuality of marriage. Homosexuality is not God's perfect will for men and women. It is unnatural.

"When we consider the causes of homosexuality, we find the road is not so simple. We have to talk about destructive home life. We have to recognize that weak, indifferent fathers and domineering mothers also fall short of God's intended purpose, whether their children fall into homosexuality or not. Most homosexuals have parents who don't know how to purposefully express their sexuality. The father failed to be the man God intended him to be; the woman fell short of God's design for her womanhood.

"This doesn't mean that the product of such a home has to be a homosexual. Most don't turn out that way.

"The biblical view also compels us to ask how God feels about homosexuals as persons. The answer is that He loves them and desires them to repent as He does all other sinners. Christ died for their sins too. None of us can be selfrighteous here.

"We hear that homosexuals can't change. They can if they want to badly enough and have the spiritual resources of faith and the Christian community. Every psychiatric study of homosexual conversion emphasizes the role of the will. For the homosexual who desires to repent and receive Christ, God's Spirit will help him find deliverance.

"The condition of latent homosexuality may still remain, just as an alcoholic who becomes a Christian may remain an alcoholic. Both need a strong affirmative Christian fellowship to keep from lapsing back into their old ways.

"Now we come to a different area of concern: How are we to deal with homosexuals in our society?

"The Mosaic Law decreed that homosexuals caught in the act were to be stoned to death. That was under a theocracy. We don't live under such a system, although our laws are to some degree rooted in the Bible.

"Colonial America was more theocratic than present society. There were criminal penalties for not attending church, for failing to pay the local ministry, and for sexual misconduct, including homosexual acts. There came a gradual awareness that religion was not the state's business. Church and state were separated, and the First Amendment to the Constitution begins, 'Congress shall make no law respecting an establishment of religion. . . .'

"Nobody suggested that all of the laws relating to religion be thrown out. Theologians and politicians talked about two tables of the Ten Commandments. The first four, they said, were religious and in the province of the church. The last six related to public order and were in the interest of the state.

"In the second division, the laws against murder, theft, and perjury are still considered necessary. But the feeling has grown that sexual relations—homosexual and heterosexual—between consenting adults outside of marriage, and other so-called "victimless" crimes should not be punished. What consenting adults do in privacy is their own business, many people say, and the state should keep its nose out.

"This rationale isn't consistently held. It's illegal to try to commit suicide. It's against the law to kill someone at his request. There are also laws against using illegal drugs.

"Because of the increase in all types of crime and the rise in permissiveness, it's becoming harder to enforce every law. Police will no longer pick up all the drunks, unless they're a public nuisance. With sexual acts, there's the problem of the right of privacy. Courts are taking a lot of interest in that today.

"At a meeting of our Christian Legal Society in California, one of our speakers, a seminary professor, took the position that penalties should be removed for homosexual acts between consenting adults. This, he said, would neither approve nor disapprove of homosexuality. It would simply say the law is not going to get involved.

"There is a reasonable limit on the imposition of law. I see no reason why homosexuals should be discriminated against in most employment. General Motors shouldn't be able to fire the guy who tightens the third bolt on a left rear fender for being gay. It doesn't interfere with his work. But I don't think that acknowledged homosexuals should teach in public schools. This is the point that Anita Bryant is making.

"In Washington State, a known homosexual was dismissed from teaching. By refusing to hear an appeal, the Supreme Court upheld the dismissal. I think the Court recognizes that a good section of the American public, more than just evangelical Christians, is strongly opposed to an avowed gay teaching homosexuality as a legitimate, alternative lifestyle in the public schools, particularly in the elementary grades.

"I would argue that a school teacher has a duty to reflect the values of the community. There is a fiduciary or trust responsibility in public education, particularly to parents who don't have the alternative of sending their children to private schools.

"The militant gays claim this is a violation of their civil rights. It seems to me that to let them have their way would violate the rights of disapproving parents.

"The gay lifestyle is really being pushed. The number of television programs in which homosexuals are presented in neutral, or even positive roles, has drastically increased. I saw one the other night where a male homosexual got engaged to a girl and then decided he had too much integrity to marry her. He said, 'I have to learn to accept myself, and quit trying to be something I'm not.' That has an impact.

"For some persons, falling into the gay system is an elective process. Influential persons are helping them to make that choice, while the view that homosexuality is abnormal and destructive is hardly heard at all. I expect this kind of permissiveness to increase.

" 'Why doesn't the law do something?' you say. Or, 'Why can't we pass a law that will keep gays from positions of influence?' Maybe this could have been done a century ago. Since then we've seen the law severed from revealed morality.

"The classic quote on this is from Justice Oliver Wendell Holmes: 'The law is not a brooding, omnipresence in the sky.' That represents, in a sense, the judicial perspective that the law is not 'out there' to find, but that we make it. In previous centuries, even people who didn't believe in a Christian, personal Deity, felt God was out there in the sense of justice.

"The primary effect of this separation has been on morality. Yet in certain areas we've seen a growing sensitivity to certain moral values—consumer rights and the civil rights of racial and ethnic minorities, for instance. In these areas, people are saying, 'Our laws ought to reflect values,' and I agree. They're talking about laws which to some extent are not up to the people, laws which represent fundamental rights. At the same time they say the law can't get involved with private sexual morality. They say there is not enough consensus to demand it. In many instances, the framers of the law don't agree with the morality the law once represented.

"England has been caught up in this same revolution, except the gay rights issue hit there before here. Lord Devlin, an influential English legal scholar, argued that some moral rules and practices are so built into the fabric of a society that their observance is critical. Society, Lord Devlin maintained, is a 'community of ideas,' to try to distinguish between public and private morality is misleading and false. His principle for defining immorality for the purpose of law is simple: 'that which every right-minded person presumes to be immoral.'

"Devlin didn't argue from a base of divine revelation. He said that some moral standards are basic to the structure of society.

"We hear it said that you can't legislate morality. That's an echo from those who once opposed integration and discriminated against blacks. Government is already legislating morality in human rights, integration, and business and corporate ethics. Morality can be changed to a degree by law, even though human nature may remain the same. Change depends on what moral practices society wants changed.

"Our society is becoming more pluralistic. The evangelical Christian ethos is no longer dominant in most localities. There is a vocal and influential minority of people who say that homosexuality is all right. Will we abdicate our responsibilities and let this view prevail in government, entertainment, and the media? As citizens of an earthly kingdom as well as a heavenly kingdom, I don't think we can back away. We have responsibilities to the society in which we live.

"How can we participate in the making and enforcing of laws against homosexual infringements on our rights and the good of society? Not by standing on our heels and screaming about moral decay in America, but by taking an active role in politics. We can support informed, committed Christian candidates. Some of us can run for office, serve on city councils and in county administrations, and be elected to legislatures. We can play a part in the legal process, even though we may not get everything we want.

"*Compromise* is a dirty word to many Christians who think of it only in theological terms. *We need to support a concept of legitimate compromise in the public arena. We ought to be in there pitching and not just squawking about our values.* We should be willing to take flak from friend and foe, and respond to the challenge of the gays."

11
Dilemmas in Dying

In the old days, the doctor would slowly walk from the bedroom of a dying family member to solemnly tell the waiting, anxious loved ones, "I've done all I can. Gather the family."

Families lived closer together then. By sunset the close relatives were there, the closest kin tiptoeing in and out of Grandma's room, where Grandpa sat holding her thin hand. The children were waiting in the yard, watching the neighbors coming with baskets of food and offers to care for the little ones while their parents kept the deathwatch.

As the night wore on and Grandma's breathing became more labored and her pulse slower, the doctor remained, unless an emergency took him away. When his sensitive fingers and ears could no longer detect her vital signs, he held a feather or mirror before her mouth to test for exhalation, then checked for reflexes. Assured that life was gone, he slowly pulled the sheet over her head and turned to console the relatives before climbing into his buggy and going home for much-needed sleep.

The rest of the death ritual was predictable. Compassionate women washed and dressed the body, and the men built a wooden coffin and dug the grave. The funeral followed at the meeting house or at the old homestead, with the loved ones freely expressing their sorrow, while the farmer-preacher stood by benevolently. Then the coffin was gently placed in a wagon and transported to the graveyard for the simple interment. Afterward, the family and close friends returned to the house for a meal and sharing of fond remembrances about Grandma. The next day the routines of life returned to normal.

That was the experience of dying when life was simpler and shorter than today, when families and neighbors were closer, when doctors were implicitly trusted and malpractice suits unthought of, when electronic medicine and miracle life-extending drugs were far into the future.

Dying Today

Barring accidents and unpredictable diseases, today's Grandma lives years longer. She usually dies in a hospital, her last days extended by the marvels of medical science, her senses mercifully dulled by pain-killing narcotics. Then she is taken to a funeral home for embalming and cosmetology. After being viewed by loved ones at a brief funeral in a portable chapel, she is efficiently buried in an expensive velvet-lined casket.

Doctors, nurses, and undertakers are professionals doing their jobs, with payment coming from insurance companies. And should the family believe that Grandma did not receive the best treatment, they may talk to lawyers. No longer is the doctor a "holy man" in society. No longer can he take the goodwill of his clientele for granted. He wonders about each patient: *Will the family sue me if my treatment is unsatisfactory to them?* He is especially concerned about what he does or fails to do for a dying patient.

Malpractice insurance is skyrocketing. Million-dollar settlements are not unusual. A Houston jury, for example, returned a nine million dollar verdict against a hospital for a fatal error in making an oxygen hookup.

For good or bad, court litigation has spotlighted a plethora of troubling issues relating to dying that never before existed:

- When is a terminally ill patient dead?
- How much treatment should a person receive during his last days? When should life support be withdrawn?
- Should doctors hasten the death process when the terminal patient is in dire pain? Should the wishes of a dying person, as expressed in a living will, be honored?
- Are laws permitting *euthanasia* (Greek: *eu*—"good," *thanatos*— "death") ever desirable? Should a doctor, nurse, or loved one be exonerated from guilt, in putting to death an incurable sufferer?
- When support resources are limited, how is a doctor to decide which of his patients shall live?

When and What is Death?

Death, in the Bible, most often means "giving up breath" (translated "ghost" in King James). It is also the dissolving, the taking down of the earthly tabernacle (2 Tim. 4:6), and the "body without the spirit" (James 2:26).

Death further marks the separation of the material from the nonmaterial part of man, the severance of man as soul from temporal relationships with earthly and physical things, and the departure of the *real* man which is soul or spirit. Theologians have attempted to explain this mystery and to define the eternal self which leaves the body. Dr. James Oliver Buswell, Jr. speaks of the "two substantive entities which make up the whole man: (1) the body, which at death returns to dust, awaiting the resurrection, and (2) the nonmaterial self which, if regenerate, goes to paradise or heaven; if not, to the abode of the wicked dead" (*Zondervan Pictorial Dictionary*, Zondervan Publishing House, p. 807).

The definition in *Webster's Seventh New Collegiate Dictionary* is deceptively simple: "a permanent cessation of all vital functions: the end of life." The problem is that vital functions do not all die at the same time.

Dr. Maurice Rawlings, author of the bestselling *Beyond Death's*

Door, distinguishes between clinical and biological death: "Clinical death occurs when the heart stops and breathing ceases, and is often reversible. Biological death is when *all* tissues have degenerated beyond function and are not reversible by medical science."

Dr. Rawlings frequently teaches classes in resuscitation. He estimates that more than 50 percent of all sudden deaths, not involving catastrophic injury, can be reversed by proper resuscitation. All hospital personnel are familiar with "Code Blue" or "Code Alert" which brings a cardiopulmonary resuscitation team on the run. The record for such restoration may be held by businessman Ben Strong of Alexandria, Louisiana. He was "brought back" 29 times in one day by the use of a defibrillator.

Speed is critical in bringing back a patient whose heart and breathing capacity have failed. According to Dr. Roger Veith, a Chattanooga neurosurgeon, the brain can survive only about three-and-one-half minutes without oxygenated blood. Brain death cannot be reversed.

The establishment of the time of legal death can be critically important in court. A husband and wife perish in a common disaster. Who dies first can make a difference in deciding inheritance rights.

The time of death can also be crucial where the violent death of a transplant donor is in dispute. In one case on record, David Potter was admitted to an English hospital suffering multiple skull fractures and extensive brain damage from a beating. After he stopped breathing, a respirator was hooked up and in two operations, 24 hours apart—as previously arranged—his kidneys were removed and transplanted. At the trial of the victim's assailant, the defense attorney blamed the removal of the vital organs for the victim's death. The examining pathologist and a neurologist disagreed, contending that the respirator had been hooked up *after* death occurred and only for the removal of the kidneys. The jury agreed with the doctors and convicted the assailant of manslaughter.

What the doctor actually records on the death certificate, notes Dr. Christopher M. Reilly, a past president of the Christian Medical Society, is the time at which the patient is pronounced dead. The trend in medicine is to follow criteria presented by Harvard University researchers in 1968: no spontaneous respiration, no reflexive response to external stimuli or to pain; a flat EEG brain wave, checked by two observers 24 hours apart when there is doubt.

There are rare instances where a flat brain wave may fall short of defining death. The American EEG Society admits that in one group of 2,650 patients declared brain dead, three later recovered some cerebral functions. All three suffered from massive overdose of nervous system depressants. The death of brain-damaged children is also sometimes difficult to establish. A Canadian physician recalls declaring one grossly handicapped boy dead four times. He now puts on the death certificate for a brain-damaged child that death occurred between such and such a time.

Where brain death is not recognized by law, doctors are understandably hesitant about performing transplants, because they have resulted in the deaths of persons who otherwise might have survived.

How Much Treatment Should a Dying Person Receive?

Dr. Reilly notes that an ethical physician has only two options in treating the terminally ill patient:

• Active treatment for maximum lengthening of life.
• Passive management to shorten the dying process.

A third alternative, euthanasia or active intervention to end life, is not permissible.

The physician must weigh the following options against a variety of factors, in consultation with colleagues, the family, and the patient if he is rational:

• The remote possibility of recovery and/or remission and the likelihood that a cure might be found if vital functions are prolonged.
• The level of pain. The ancient Hippocratic oath binds the doctor to do all possible to relieve pain and lengthen life. But the modern doctor is often unable to relieve pain without shortening life.
• The financial impact on the family for further doubtful treatment. Will the cost, often running over $50,000, be adequately covered by insurance? Will the bill put the family in a bind for years to come?
• The use of medical care and equipment which might otherwise be provided for a patient with a better prognosis.

- Legal questions where a doctor may be afraid to discontinue "extraordinary" treatment for fear of being sued.
- Life quality. When does a dying patient reach the point where his vital functions are not worth maintaining?

Guidelines vary from one hospital to another. Staff physicians in smaller institutions tend to have a mutual understanding about when to use extraordinary life support. They will not give oxygen support from a ventilator to a patient who is dying of lung cancer. Nor will they try to resuscitate someone hopelessly ill with heart disease.

Larger hospitals, such as Mt. Sinai in New York City, tend to be more explicit in instructions to staff. Four levels of care are established at Mt. Sinai's Falk Surgical-Respiratory Intensive Care Unit.

Every patient coming into intensive care is placed on Level 1 and given full life support. If evaluation indicates a chance of survival, he remains on this level.

If his chances are deemed remote, he is dropped to Level 2. Here he receives the same treatment as at the upper level, but his condition is reevaluated every 24 hours. If he shows improvement, he goes back to Level 1. If he worsens, he may be downgraded to Level 3.

Level 3 is for patients with no measurable chance of survival. No new treatment is initiated here. Patients receive comfort care only, no blood transfusions if they hemorrhage, no antibiotics if infections develop, no resuscitation if they go into cardiac arrest. Only two "miracle" patients placed on this level have ever recovered.

Level 4 is for the brain dead. All life support is discontinued. Patients remain until enough time has elapsed for them to be declared legally dead.

Dying Goes to Court

Headline-making court battles follow the removal of life support, usually a respirator which helps the patient breathe. The most sensational is the Karen Quinlan case.

Depressed over her own drug addiction, and rejection by a boyfriend, the 21-year-old woman took 140 tranquilizers and tried to drive her car into a stone wall. She was taken, in a coma, to a hospital in Denville, New Jersey and placed on a respirator. In "a chronic vegetative state" (words of her doctors) she was kept on the machine for a year while her permanently damaged brain continued to emit steady though slight signals on an EEG machine.

The parents asked for the respirator to be removed. The doctors refused, and the case went to court. Medical experts disagreed on the witness stand, and Catholic theologians opposed one another. Finally the New Jersey State Supreme Court gave Miss Quinlan's stepfather the right to obtain other doctors who would be willing to unplug the respirator. She was taken off the mechanical respirator in June, but left on intravenous feedings and antibiotics. The case was called a landmark. Never before had a court made a decision intended to result in the removal of life support.

Three years after the respirator was taken away, Karen Quinlan is still alive. She lies comatose and curled in a fetal position in a nursing home. Her parents faithfully visit her every day, but she shows no sign of recognition.

What Is Euthanasia?

Is withholding extraordinary life support really passive euthanasia? The doctors we interviewed unanimously said No. The attending physician is simply letting an irreversible disease take its natural course.

After extraordinary support is stopped, the terminal patient usually has but a short time to live. At this point the doctor may, after consulting with the family, and the patient, if rational, increase the dosage and frequency of pain-killing narcotics. Comfort is exchanged for a few extra days of painful life. The sufferer dies in dignity without feeling pain.

Doctors admit this is on the borderline between passive management to shorten the dying process and active intervention to end life. But no physician has ever been convicted of a crime for making a patient "comfortable" in his last hours.

Euthanasia generates controversy and concern. If another person— the doctor, nurse, or family member—ends the patient's life, a homicide charge can result. If the patient kills himself, it is suicide, and may affect the payout of his insurance. In the few such homicide cases that have gone to court, juries have not been eager to convict.

The classic defendant is Dr. Hermann N. Sanders of Hillsboro, New Hampshire. In 1949 he was charged with murdering a 59-year-old woman cancer patient by injecting air into her veins.

Dr. Sanders testified in court that the woman's husband had constantly begged him to do something about her suffering. The doctor further said that he was worried about the husband's bad heart. He freely admitted injecting the air on impulse, to make certain that she experienced no more pain. However, an expert defense witness from Harvard Medical School attributed the patient's death to natural causes. The jury returned a verdict of Not Guilty.

In March 1979, a Baltimore nurse, Mary Rose Robaczynski, was accused of disconnecting the life support systems of four comatose GORK (short for "God Only Really Knows" if they are dead or alive) patients. She was first tried for allegedly killing Harry Gessner, 48, a Baltimore taxi driver, who after suffering heart failure was resuscitated and moved to the special care unit of Maryland General Hospital where the defendant worked. The defense argued that the patient was already dead when the respirator was disconnected. The prosecution said he was still alive. The jury deadlocked on a verdict and the judge declared a mistrial. At this writing, dates for new trials on the deaths of the four patients are pending.

Katie Roberts, a hopeless invalid from muscular dystrophy, tried and failed to commit suicide by taking carbolic acid. She then asked her husband to mix a poison and place it on a chair near her bed. This time she was successful. However, a Michigan jury declared him guilty of murder in the first degree and sentenced him to life imprisonment.

In a similar case, Mrs. Alice Waskin, a Chicago leukemia victim, tried to end her pain with an overdose of sleeping pills. Saved in a hospital emergency room, she was admitted to an intensive-care unit. There her 24-year-old son, Robert, kissed her and fired two bullets into her head. A jury found him not guilty by reason of temporary insanity.

A husband and wife, both incurably ill, may make a suicide pact. Dr. Henry Pitney Van Dusen was a leading liberal Protestant churchman, seminary president, and one of the founders of the World Council of Churches. A stroke left him unable to speak or write. His wife suffered from severe arthritis.

They took an overdose of sleeping pills and she died. He vomited up the pills but died two weeks later from a heart ailment.

A terminally ill patient may ask a doctor to provide a lethal weapon in drugs. Dr. Nathan Schanaper, a Baltimore psychiatrist, told of an incurable who bargained for a sizable amount of barbiturates for "when the time comes." The doctor told a reporter, "I might end up handing him 50 Seconal and say, 'One a night; it's to help you sleep.' But he knows what to do with Seconal. . . . Morally," Dr. Schanaper asks, "Is it more difficult to let somebody die an obscene, undignified, miserable, painful death? Or to help him in some way to die quickly, when you know he has to die?" (*Washington Post*, March 12, 1974)

The Euthanasia Society of America, formed in 1935 under the leadership of Unitarian Minister Charles Francis Potter, proposes to allow a court to receive a petition from the attending physician diagnosing a disease as incurable. The court would then appoint a commission of three, including two doctors, to investigate and report back. If the commission recommended and the court approved, then the physician could take measures to end the incurable's life. Such a law has never passed a single state legislature. The idea is strenuously opposed by evangelical theologians.

A similar group in England proposes that certain forms of mercy killing be made a "minor offense" and apply to persons who from compassion unlawfully kill someone believed to be in great pain or permanently helpless from physical or mental incapacity. Such a law is strongly opposed by the organization, Nationwide Festival of Light, formed in 1971 by evangelical Christians to fight against the decline in public and private morals. Previously, the British Parliament, with loud cries of "No, No, No!" rejected a measure that would have permitted a person to exercise his own choice in death.

Euthanasia efforts in Denmark, Sweden, and Switzerland have also made no headway. There has been no public effort in France and Italy because of the strong influence of the Catholic Church which vigorously opposes euthanasia. In West Germany the subject is almost unmentionable because of revulsion against the Nazi program of ending 70,000 "worthless lives"—mostly crippled and mentally defective persons.

Most leading physicians throughout Western society oppose any law that would give even the medical profession sanction to actively intervene and end life. "Give the physician too much power, and it can be abused," warns Dr. Edmund Pellegrino, Professor of Medicine at Yale University (*U.S. News and World Report,* November 3, 1975, p. 53).

Is There a Right to Die?

The so-called "right-to-die" movement has been gaining momentum. One thrust is to promote "Living Wills" which are witnessed, notarized, and addressed to "my family, clergyman, physician, and lawyer, for a time when I may be incapable of deciding my own future." The key paragraph usually requests,

If there is no reasonable expectation of my recovering from an illness or injury, I request that I be allowed to die in dignity and not be kept alive by heroic measures. I ask that drugs be administered to me only for the relief of pain and not to prolong my earthly life, even if these pain-killing drugs may hasten my death.

Most doctors, according to an American Medical Association poll, will honor such instructions, although they are not legally bound to do so.

Who Shall Live?

This is perhaps the most difficult decision of all. The most rare example is the choice doctors must make in separating Siamese twins who share a heart (once in 100,000 births). In October 1977, Philadelphia lawyers went to court to defend surgeons who had been asked to separate Siamese babies joined at the chest. The lawyers reasoned that no homicide occurs if an act is done under a court order, where the good anticipated from the act would outweigh the bad. They cited an argument from a rabbi about two mountain climbers hanging from a ledge that would only support one. The rabbi said the climber with the more secure hold was justified in cutting his partner's rope.

The court ordered that the three-month-old babies should be separated and that the one designated by the surgeons as stronger should keep the heart.

Much more frequent is a situation where the director of a hospital intensive care unit must decide to move out one critically ill patient to make room for another who is younger and has a better chance. It also happens when only one organ for transplant is available and two patients are waiting. Who will die without it? A hospital committee often makes this choice.

Some authorities see a much larger dilemma looming in the future, with the population of the elderly increasing to a critical point. A British doctor, John Goundry, predicts that a "death pill" for old people will be available and perhaps obligatory within 20 years. Dr. Goundry wrote in the magazine *Pulse* for British physicians: "Society's view of life will change from the sentimental to the calculated and sophisticated, and the overriding policy will be the survival of the fittest." Dr. Goundry finds it puzzling that "we now have a science which stops people from being born (abortion), and the meddlesome science of geriatrics which stops us from dying." An official of the British National Federation of Old Persons responded: "The sick and infirm need looking after, not killing off. I hope this pill comes to him some day" (August 6, 1977).

In juxtaposing euthanasia with abortion, the Englishman is not alone. Asks Joseph Fletcher, progenitor of modern situation ethics: "Why is fetal euthanasia all right, but not terminal euthanasia?" (*Christianity Today*, November 21, 1975, p. 36)

12

Christian Perspectives on Dilemmas in Dying

DR. CARL WENGER, GENERAL SURGEON

"Treatment of a terminally ill patient," the Little Rock surgeon admits, "is a sticky problem. This is emphasized by the fact that the courts are having such a time defining death.

"What makes it even more difficult is that people are becoming volitionally programmed in our society to the thought that it is immoral to die. As a result, the physician is often open to criticism if he doesn't use 'heroics' to prolong what is called *life*. But how do you define *life* at various stages in the dying process?

"I am personally much interested in what Jesus said in John 17:3: 'And this is eternal life, that they may know Thee, the only true God, and Jesus Christ whom Thou hast sent.' I take this principle of 'knowing' and apply to the dying patient. If I have someone who can communicate and reciprocate love with his family, I will continue to support that patient with extraordinary means as long as he 'knows', even though the end can't be far off. He may not even be able to talk, but I'll still give him support. I've known instances where the pressure of a hand on the hand of a loved one has been a real source of comfort. That to me is the name of the game, being able to know and be known."

Dr. Wenger never makes an important decision alone on the care of a terminal patient. "I always enlist the family. I never put a patient on the respirator except with their concurrence. I tell them death is imminent and ask if they want heroic measures. They often ask, 'Doctor, what do you think?' I tell them that in my judgment we will gain little from it. Generally, we decide together not to put the loved one on a respirator, not to attempt to resuscitate when vital signs fail.

"It's unusual for a family not to concur with my judgment. I deal more with terminal cancer patients than with any other group, and rarely find a family that wants to protract the misery that almost inevitably comes with cancer death.

"It's hard, terribly hard, for a family to concede the imminent death of a loved one. I remember a mother dying with inoperable cancer of the pancreas. When she began to bleed from her tumor, I told the family, 'We have two options: One, we can give blood and try to prolong life. Two, we can not give blood and recognize that in a few hours her blood pressure will go down and she will die.' One of the sons said, 'Doctor, can't we give her just a little blood?' He was reluctant to take the responsibility for not giving any help, but he didn't want his mother to suffer anymore. So we did just that. He was at peace. He didn't have to live with the decision that he had played a part in causing his mother's death, and by the same token he didn't have to watch her suffer for a protracted length of time."

Dr. Wenger believes in being absolutely truthful with the family and the patient. "I don't go out of the way to answer questions that haven't been asked. But I always answer questions.

"Sometimes, after surgery, the patient will say, 'What did you find, Doc?' 'We found a growth,' I'll say. Some will ask right then, 'Was it cancer?' and I'll tell them it was. If they don't ask, I don't tell them. A week later, I'll be making rounds, and a patient will say, 'Doc, sit down. We haven't really talked about what you did, and what I have. I want it straight.' So we go over the details. I'll answer questions, give statistics, be frank. After that if he asks me, 'How am I doing?' I can tell him, and he'll believe me.

"I've had patients say, 'Doctor, I know I have cancer, but don't tell my family.' And the family will say, 'We know Dad has cancer, but don't tell him.' Here the physician is denying the family one of the most tremendous experiences in the whole spectrum of human experience, facing a crisis together, supporting one another. I tell a family that doesn't want their loved one to know: 'There'll come a time when your father is going to need all the support we can give him. He will learn sooner or later the truth. If we lie to him at this point, when another crisis arises he'll wonder if we're lying then. When he really needs support he will have legitimate doubt in his mind about whether this support is valid.' They usually go along.

"Still, I've had some flatly tell me, 'We don't want him to know!' So I'll tell the patient, 'Your family has asked me not to discuss your illness with you.' That tells him what he wants to know and I haven't betrayed the family. I just tell him, 'You talk with your family; I've given them all the details.' "

Dr. Wenger believes a patient's wish to die in dignity should be honored. "My brother, the president of a Christian college, died about two years ago. He had a coronary and lived just a week. Arthur told his wife, 'If this is my time, I don't want the tubes all over me.' They respected his request.

"If a patient makes a rational decision when faced with a crisis, I'll go along with him. I had a woman come into the hospital recently. 'I don't want any tubes or IVs,' she said. 'I'm a believer in the Lord Jesus Christ, I know I'm going to die, and I want it that way.' I documented on the record that in my judgment the patient was lucid, rational, terminal, and the family was in complete agreement. I was there on a daily basis, made every provision for her comfort, and let the disease take its natural course.

"I remember another woman patient who also happened to have cancer of the pancreas. A nurse asked her, 'Aren't you afraid to stay alone?' She said, 'I'm not alone! I sense the presence of the Lord, as I never have. Don't worry about me.' To invade that consciousness with a lot of physical activity, and to deprive this little lady of what she recognized not as a terminus but a transition, would have been wrong. Now if she'd been afraid and wanted support, I'd have gone along with her in a minute."

This isn't passive euthanasia, in Dr. Wenger's viewpoint. "I'm simply permitting an irreversible disease to take its natural course. I don't become aggressive. I give pain killers. I'll give intravenous fluids to a patient unable to eat. But when the pressure begins to fall, I don't try to bring it up, and when respiration begins to fail, I don't put him on a respirator. However, if there's any potential for reversing the situation, I pull out all the stops.

"The dying patient needs to know that the doctor cares. I think that many times what is interpreted as rudeness and disinterest on the part of the physician is really a defense. He knows involvement with the terminally ill is emotionally draining. The doctor may also be afraid, apprehensive, not only about death but about being asked for spiritual advice. So many, many times, I've heard a physician say, 'I hate to go in that room.'

"The Christian physician can give special comfort. I'm not given to taking advantage of a situation, but I frequently tell of my personal faith. This often leads to a sigh of relief from the family and the patient, if he can communicate. 'We're glad you feel that way,' they'll often say, 'because we do too.'

"Some Christians are afraid to express their emotions. They feel it is a mark of weakness. I don't believe that. Jesus wept when He heard of the death of Lazarus. Christ in His humanity had experienced the trauma of separation from a man He really loved. I tell families that it is not a mark of their inadequacy, or a lack of faith in God, to express their feelings.

"Sometimes I'll have a patient, in our death-denying society, who is better prepared than the family or even the medical attendants. One day I was making rounds with a medical student and came to the bedside of a little lady covered with tubes. 'You know, I can hardly wait,' she murmured. 'What do you mean?' I asked. 'I just want to be with the Lord,' she said.

"When we slipped out, I told the student, 'I sort of envy her.' 'What do you mean?' he asked. I looked at him. 'How many decisions have you ever made predicated on the fact that you are going to die someday? Probably you buy life insurance, and that's because some guy knocks on your door.' He had to agree. 'Here's a little lady who makes every decision considering that she's going to die soon. You know that would give your decisions a quality they are not going to have any other way.' He looked at me, then just turned his head. He didn't quite know how to handle it."

DR. MAURICE RAWLINGS, CARDIOVASCULAR SPECIALIST

Dr. Rawlings' research for his best-selling book, *Beyond Death's Door*, and his conversion to Christ were spurred by a rural mail carrier's experience after death. The carrier fell dead while Dr. Rawlings was performing a "stress test" to evaluate complaints of chest pains. Each time Dr. Rawlings and assisting nurses resuscitated him, he would scream, "I am in hell! Don't stop!"

"He had a terrified look, worse than the expression normally seen in death," Dr. Rawlings recalls. "His pupils were dilated, and he was perspiring and trembling—he looked as if his hair was on end. . . . After several such death episodes, he finally asked me, 'How do I stay out of hell?' I told him, 'I guess it's the same principle you learned in Sunday School. I guess Jesus Christ is the One you would ask to save you.'

"Then he said, 'I don't know how. Pray for me.' I knew I had no choice. It was a dying man's request. So I had him repeat a prayer after me as we worked—right there on the floor."

The patient's condition finally stabilized and Dr. Rawlings put him in a hospital. Convinced that there really was life after death, Dr. Rawlings dusted off his Bible and sought more understanding. Through the experience, the once skeptical physician and the mail carrier both accepted Christ.

From this point on, Dr. Rawlings began interviewing resuscitated patients. He found that about 20 percent had something to tell. After a few interviews he also realized that his research differed from accounts by Dr. Elisabeth Kubler-Ross and other physician-authors on experiences of resuscitated patients. The other writers recorded mostly pleasant experiences. Some of Dr. Rawlings' informants, like the mail carrier, told of being near or actually in hell. The explanation, Dr. Rawlings decided, was that he had interviewed patients as soon as possible after resuscitation, while their memories were still clear, while the other doctors had waited months, and in some cases over a year.

Could these experiences just beyond death's door be the mind playing tricks, since the brain was still alive?

"Well, they would have to be mass hallucinations," Dr. Rawlings says. "Everybody getting on the phone to one another, coming to the same conclusion. They don't all have the identical story, but they do have the same sequence. Also a few show recall of what actually went on in the room while they were in the death process. They recalled sound sometimes—hearing is one of the last senses to go. A few also saw things, even though their eyes were closed."

Dr. Rawlings finds his research on life after death intriguing and compelling, and he speaks frequently on the subject. But he is also concerned about dying patients.

"Is it more important to keep a patient alive or to maintain quality of life?" he asks. "Doctors are tending to go in the latter direction now. I know I am. I try to treat the patient as if he were myself. Would I want to be kept alive a few days or weeks longer or be kept comfortable?

"I talk with the dying patient and his family about this, and if they agree, I vow with them that so long as I am the attending physician, I will see that the patient goes out without worry or pain."

Dr. Rawlings concedes that medications for comfort and pain relief speed the death process. "But this isn't a form of euthanasia," he declares. "It isn't sudden. It's just keeping them comfortable until the end comes."

He believes the court cases on treatment of dying patients have been caused "because the doctor wouldn't listen to the family. If you will just be honest with the patient and family from the beginning and say you are going to treat the patient as your own mother or yourself, then you're clear. You treat a *person* instead of a number or case. You serve the patient at his bedside with compassion.

"For me the patient's desire is first, if he's in his right mind, and then the family's. I've never needed a court order to alter medical treatment of a dying patient."

Does he favor a hospital death committee to make difficult decisions? "Not necessarily, at least not in our hospital. You get cross consultations, especially where there's a question of a terminal illness. But if you stay with the family, you can avoid too many expensive tests.

"I tell the family when bills are running up and we aren't getting anywhere. They usually suggest that we don't continue. Then instead of pulling the plug on a patient where we're using a ventilator, we gradually decrease the oxygen and the frequency of use. The idea is if he can't make it on his own, he is not living. Then we remove the support apparatus slowly and keep him comfortable, while letting him go.

"There are families who will run up bills of 20 to 30 thousand dollars, all while the doctor is saying there's no use, no help at all. I remember a nurse whose son suffered a crushing head injury in a jeep accident. We kept him on all the machinery and finally he was taken home, just a vegetable, couldn't see anybody, unconscious, having enemas for bowel movements, being fed intravenously, draining the resources of his mother. He died and now she's paying off the bills. We can't understand why she would do that. But how are you going to overrule a mother? I would hate to see some formal committee telling her she couldn't have her boy."

Like Dr. Wenger, Dr. Rawlings doesn't believe in pressuring a patient on spiritual matters. "That doesn't mean I won't level with a person, even if he has a good chance to make it. I tell him, 'Pray for the best, but I've got to tell you your chances are 50-50. It's best you be prepared, get right with God, put your financial and other personal affairs in order.'

"The dying patient, the one without a medical chance," Dr. Rawlings believes, "is the most neglected of all patients, both emotionally and spiritually. Most ministers aren't trained to take care of these needs. Doctors aren't either. The family usually won't help because they are frightened at the concept of death. They play games with the patient when he's seeking answers to questions that really bother him. He wants to know, 'Does it hurt when you die?' Nobody will tell him.

'Is there life after death? Is the Bible true or not?' He may never have cared very much before. But he does now.

"Patients like this, I find, don't want to hear from a minister. They've been programmed against religion. I had a hard-nosed judge, whom I tell about in my book, with a malignant lymphoma. He wouldn't let a minister in, but he casually asked me, 'Do you believe in life after death?' That was my cue. After several conversations, he turned to Christ.

"A newspaper man, whom I'd been treating previously for heart disease, developed cancer of the pancreas. It was inoperable and incurable and he knew it. One day he asked me privately if I believed in God. We started talking, looking at Scripture. He began changing slowly until he was always inquiring about the welfare of other people, never talking about himself. He died this way, trusting in Christ."

Dr. Rawlings yearns for more Christians to become interested in ministries to the dying. "This is a very special type of ministry. You go in ministering to needs. Introduce yourself. A church might turn them off. Say, 'I'm visiting sick patients and I just wanted to know if there's anything you need. Can I talk to you a while?' Find out where they live, their job, children, things like that. If you show interest in them, the spiritual part will come naturally.

"This ministry has been overlooked and is much neglected. I'm trying to get a corps of minister-trained laymen involved, and nurses who are trained to spot patients who are not being visited. It's important, terribly important. What could be more worthwhile than helping a terminal patient find assurance of salvation and peace with God?"

DR. A. KURT WEISS, PROFESSOR OF PHYSIOLOGY

"The dilemmas in the care of the dying are caused by the success of medical science in keeping people alive longer," Dr. Weiss says. "I don't say that's bad. A good deal of my research has been on the aging process. But should we keep people alive when their normal life span has ended? I think not.

"There's also a theological question involved here: When does the soul leave the body? Some Orthodox Jews will open a window when someone dies to let the soul depart. I frankly don't know when or how the soul departs. We are much too occupied with dogma on these points. Talk to two or three pastors and you will find that each has a different way of interpreting the same phenomenon. It may just be that the soul need not depart from the body right then and there, and that that which is invisible need not be defined by our terms anyway. My point is that when somebody comes to the end of his life, and his physicians know it, it is the end of his life. Don't drag it out.

"A Christian, of all people, shouldn't want to hang on to the old decaying flesh. Since he knows his body is corruptible, he should be looking forward to the body which will not be subject to decay, a body like Christ's resurrected body. That's my hope.

"But we still have to be concerned about the here and now. To me, a much bigger problem than extending life or fighting over when to pull the plug is this: How are we going to care for the increasing number of old people who, thanks to medical science, are living longer than they would have 50 years ago? People are forced to retire from their primary vocation and they think they're at the end of life. We need to help our retirees find a second, useful occupation, and help Christian seniors develop a gift of ministry.

"Inevitably, there does come a time when a person is unable to live independently. He may be physically or mentally incapacitated, or both. As recently as 150 years ago in Vienna, Austria you could pay about a dollar on Sunday afternoon to visit the lunatic asylum and see the inmates standing there in catatonia or making silly faces. Today we have hospitals for people who are physically or mentally acutely ill. What we don't have is adequate nursing care facilities for the larger number of persons who can't be on their own but don't require a hospital bed.

"This includes many of the terminally ill. They need to be in a place of tender, loving care, a place not as expensive as the hospital, where they can die in peace. That type of place, a hospice, is presently available in only a very few localities.

"Let me summarize. Medically we've progressed. We've extended the life span about as far as we can go, I think. The psychosocial and the economic situations are where our primary concern should now be put."

DR. ROGER VEITH, NEUROSURGEON:

"Not a week goes by that I don't have to deal with the question of how much support to give a terminal patient," says Dr. Veith. "Usually it's someone with extensive brain damage. I make sure he is able to breathe without any obstruction. If he has a fever, say pneumonia, then I treat the pneumonia, and if he has a bleeding problem, I'll try to stop the bleeding. But if he has difficulty breathing because of extensive brain damage, I don't make him breathe. If his blood pressure drops because he is terminal, I don't put him on medication to maintain blood pressure. I just don't interfere with the normal body processes when I believe he will not survive, or if his chances of having any quality of life which he knew before are impossible.

"There are things worse than death. Death is very kind if you have a desperate, frightened, shaking family watching a child or loved one who is essentially dead, but living for days and days, even weeks and months, on a respirator when you know what the outcome will be. The loved ones are drained physically, emotionally, and financially. Few people can stand the cost."

In his 13 years as a neurosurgeon, Dr. Veith can recall only one case "that was without a doubt, in my judgment, a miraculous faith healing. A number of years ago I operated on a woman in her 50s who had an aneurysm, a weak spot in a blood vessel on the brain. After I clipped the aneurysm, she did extremely well and went home. About a year later she had another one. She came in very weak and I put her in intensive care. The aneurysm had already ruptured and she was bleeding—about a third of such patients die at this time. She was also decerebrate. Her pupils were fixed and there was no purposeful response when we stimulated her.

"She stayed that way for several days, absolutely nonresponsive. I moved her out of the intensive-care unit because I felt she was terminal. One night the nurse called me and said she was very bad. I went in to see her. Her respiration was labored and I thought she was going to die.

"That night and the next day she got worse and worse. Her blood pressure and pulse were dropping and she was having lots of trouble breathing. Then after she had stopped breathing, I thought, for reasons unknown to me, *I'll just do a tracheotomy* (put a small tube in her windpipe) *and make the death a little easier.* This allowed her to breathe a bit, but I told the family, 'Well, absolutely, this is the end. She'll certainly die within a day or so.'

"I came back the next morning and went over, as I always do when a patient is unconscious, and put my hand in hers and said some kind words. She squeezed my hand! I looked at her and called her name, and she opened her eyes and tried to talk to me! I had never seen something like this, and could not believe it. She went on to improve daily and a week or so later I operated on her. She recovered nicely and is still doing well.

"About a year later her husband came and asked to talk to me. He said, 'I haven't had the nerve before to tell you what happened to my wife. That night when she was so bad, our little church had an all-night prayer session. The next morning, about six, just starting daybreak, I looked up and saw Jesus at the window. He told me, "It's going to be okay." I went over to look at her, and I put my hand on her hand and she squeezed.'

"Of course, I've had other patients who were Christians whose loved ones didn't recover. You can certainly tell the difference with a family of believers. Death for them is not an everlasting defeat."